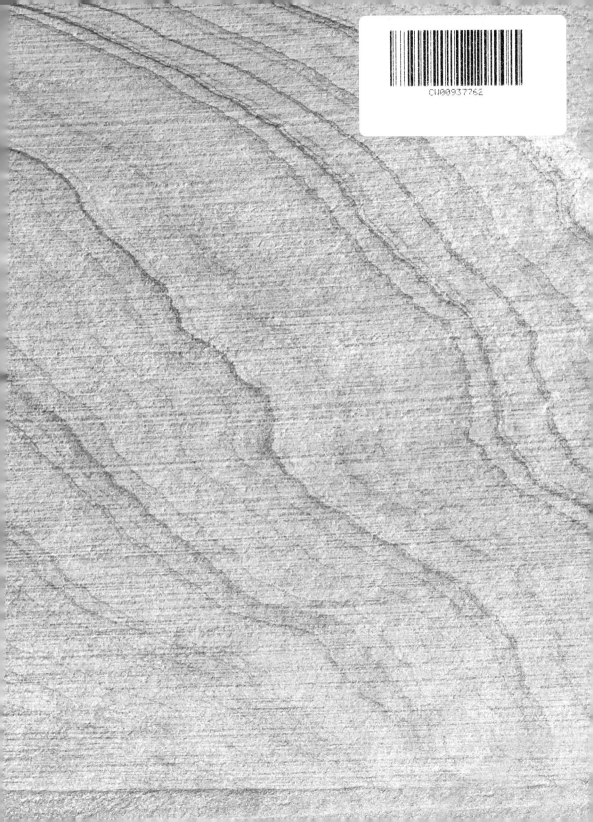

Design
a healthy
home

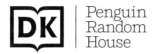

Publishing Director Katie Cowan
Art Director Maxine Pedliham
Senior Acquisitions Editor Stephanie Milner
Managing Art Editor Bess Daly
Creative direction and design Sarah Snelling
Project Editor Laura Gladwin
Designer Jordan Lambley
Editorial Assistant Kiron Gill
Jacket Designer Nicola Powling
Jackets Coordinator Lucy Philpott
Production Editor Heather Blagden
Production Controller Kariss Ainsworth

Illustrated by Sergei Tihomirov

First published in Great Britain in 2021 by
Dorling Kindersley Limited
DK, One Embassy Gardens, 8 Viaduct Gardens,
London, SW11 7BW

A CIP catalogue record for this book
is available from the British Library.
ISBN: 978-0-2415-0092-7

Printed and bound in Slovakia

For the curious
www.dk.com

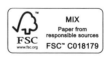

This book was made with Forest Stewardship
Council ™ certified paper – one small step
in DK's commitment to a sustainable future.
For more information go to
www.dk.com/our-green-pledge

Design a healthy home

100 ways to transform your space for physical and mental wellbeing

OLIVER HEATH

with **VICTORIA JACKSON,**

EDEN GOODE and **JO BASTON**

Contents

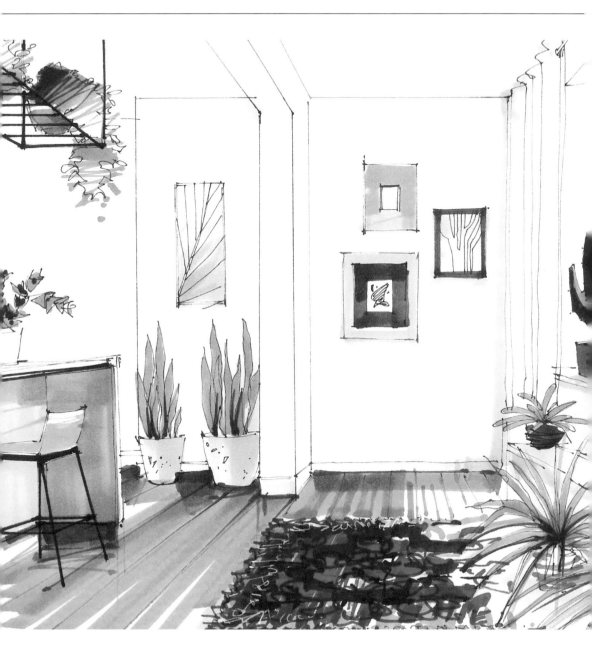

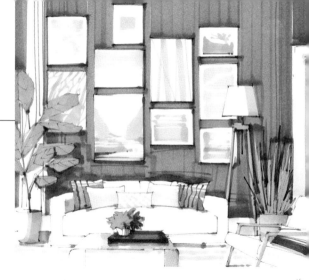

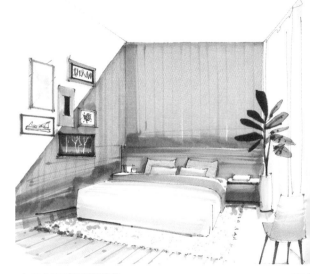

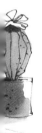

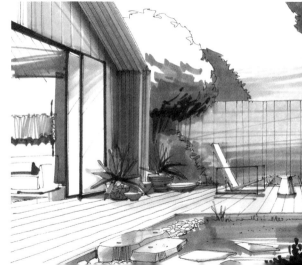

Contents

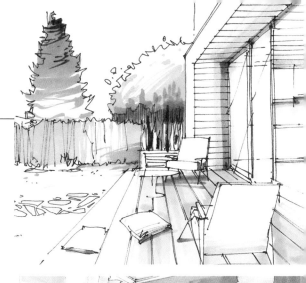

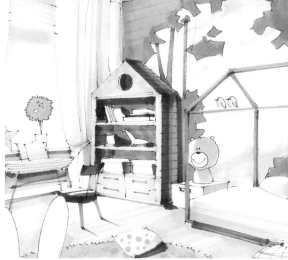

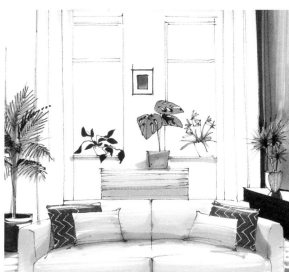

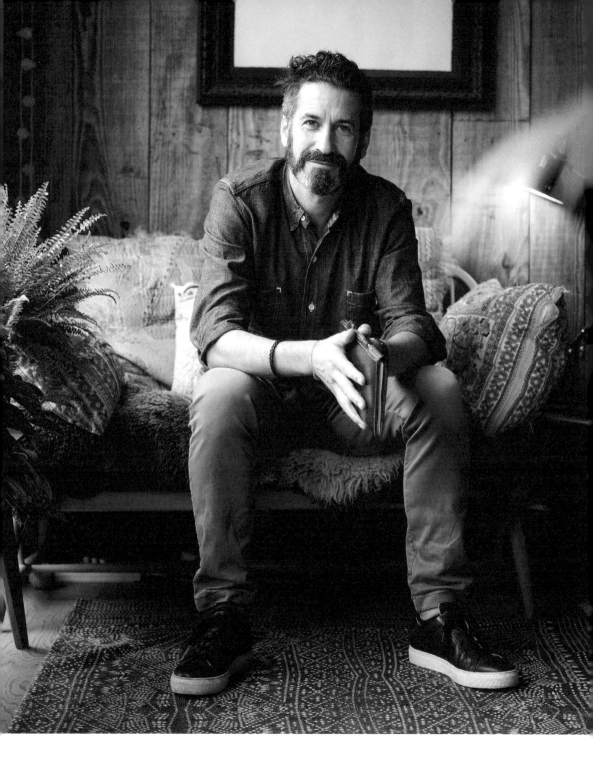

Foreword

Welcome to your starting point for creating a happier, healthier home! Like me, you've probably recognized that your home is the most important place in your life – a place that you can shape and change, and which has a real impact on how you feel about, and interact with, the world around you.

When it comes to interior design, all too often we use it as a way of expressing our identity, to show our style, status, power or wealth. These are all extrinsic, or external, considerations. What if we were to turn this around and instead take an intrinsic approach, drawing on what matters most to us, making every design choice an opportunity to improve our physical and mental wellbeing? What would it look, feel, smell or sound like? Could your home make you feel better?

Over the last eight years, I have been working with an inspirational team at Oliver Heath Design, with backgrounds in architecture, interiors, sustainable design and psychology, to uncover how the spaces we inhabit can have a deep impact on our mental, physical and emotional states. During this time, we have become thought leaders in biophilic design (more on that in a moment), writing white papers and designing strategies and spaces for world-leading organizations that have improved people's working lives through the spaces they live and work in.

Our research started in commercial design (offices, retail and educational spaces), where we had to demonstrate the value of a human-centred approach. We found that putting wellbeing first can help businesses improve their outcomes through the increased focus, productivity, and engagement of people in their buildings, as well as by reducing costs from high staff turnover and absenteeism.

It has taken longer to demonstrate the value of a human-centred approach in our homes – where a business case isn't relevant – so in the domestic sphere the movement has been slower to take off. However, with the 2020 pandemic and global lockdowns, many of us worked from home and became acutely aware of how much impact our own four walls can have on us. So we decided to take all the good stuff we've learned over the years and translate it into the home, to help people create happier, healthier places to live in.

We hope that, by exploring some of the 100 ways to create a healthier home in this book, your home can relax and restore you, help you recuperate, connect you with others and improve the quality of your life in many other ways. In each chapter we investigate key issues to tackle to improve wellbeing in your home, both practical issues such as air quality, water and temperature, and softer design issues like colour, texture, light and connection with nature. We have distilled complex issues into bite-sized pieces to introduce the things we feel you should be aware of. Each one is a good place to begin, and we encourage you to go out and investigate further.

We have tried to ensure our solutions are relevant across a range of types of home ownership and budget. Whether you're renting, buying your first home or creating a better home for you and your family, you'll find ways to improve your space and the quality of your life in it.

A biophilic design approach

Our approach to mental and physical wellbeing is based on biophilic design principles. This design ethos builds on the concept of biophilia, the innate human attraction to nature and all that is alive.

Humans' universal appreciation of nature can be traced back to long before we became urban dwellers, and makes sense when you consider that we evolved in natural settings. After all, it was out in nature that we learned how to survive and thrive; where understanding our environment and nature's cycles enabled us to flourish.

Our ancestors navigated their way through life by observing things such as sunrise, sunset, the seasons, animals, plants and weather patterns. Their senses were finely attuned to understanding these environments and it would have been crucial to recognize landscapes that could support life, to be able to differentiate between safety and danger, make quick decisions and keep fight or flight responses in full working order.

The biophilia hypothesis proposed by the biologist E O Wilson suggests that we have inherited all of this from our ancestors, and our physiology is still very much adapted to seeking a connection with nature today. We might live in noisy, crowded, busy, geometric urban spaces, but we still benefit from interacting with nature and need to remember that we are very much a part of it.

Another scientific idea, the savannah theory, suggests that we still have a preference for looking out over lush, healthy forms of nature from a point of safety. In doing so, our heart rate and blood pressure lowers, we can relax better, and we can recuperate faster from stress and exhaustion. So how do we translate these ideas into our dense urban environments and, furthermore, into our homes?

This basic evolutionary concept has been developed over the years into what we now know as biophilic design, which offers a set of three core design principles that aim to improve our connection with nature:

Nature in the space: bringing real forms of nature and ways to connect to natural systems into your space. In this book, we focus on the senses: what we can see, touch, smell, hear and taste that remind us of nature.

Natural analogues: including references to, or representations of, nature, taking inspiration from its forms, shapes, colours, patterns and textures, and even the way technology can copy them.

Nature of the space: mimicking the spatial qualities of natural environments to enhance

Our design ethos builds on the concept of biophilia, the innate human attraction to nature and all that is alive

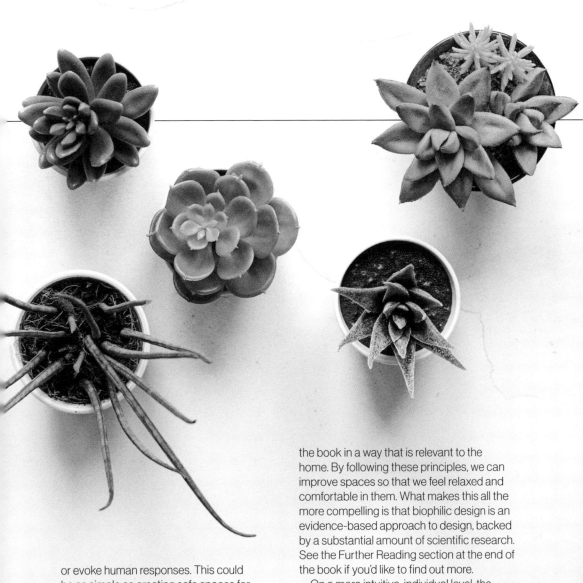

or evoke human responses. This could be as simple as creating safe spaces for retreat or configuring your space to allow for longer sightlines.

These three core principles have been developed by designers, environmental strategists and architects into a series of biophilic design practices, and we have made sure to touch on each one throughout

the book in a way that is relevant to the home. By following these principles, we can improve spaces so that we feel relaxed and comfortable in them. What makes this all the more compelling is that biophilic design is an evidence-based approach to design, backed by a substantial amount of scientific research. See the Further Reading section at the end of the book if you'd like to find out more.

On a more intuitive, individual level, the crucial thing is to draw from positive memories of being in nature and to bring that association into the home to create a beneficial response. The following 100 ways embody our approach to biophilic design in the home. We hope they inspire you to dive in and make some changes for the better!

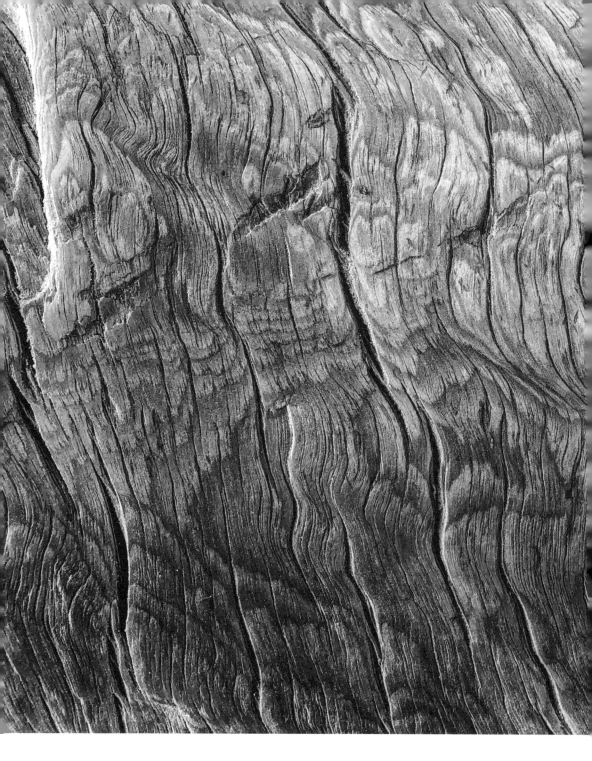

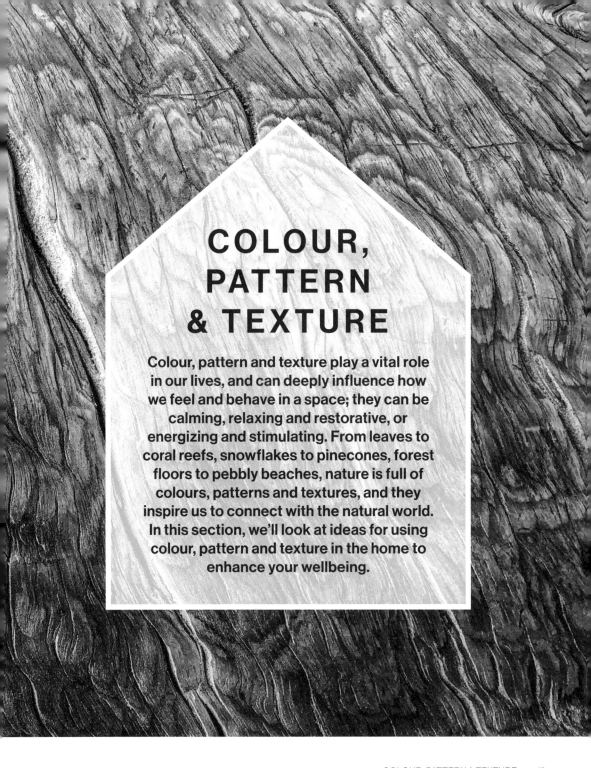

COLOUR, PATTERN & TEXTURE

Colour, pattern and texture play a vital role in our lives, and can deeply influence how we feel and behave in a space; they can be calming, relaxing and restorative, or energizing and stimulating. From leaves to coral reefs, snowflakes to pinecones, forest floors to pebbly beaches, nature is full of colours, patterns and textures, and they inspire us to connect with the natural world. In this section, we'll look at ideas for using colour, pattern and texture in the home to enhance your wellbeing.

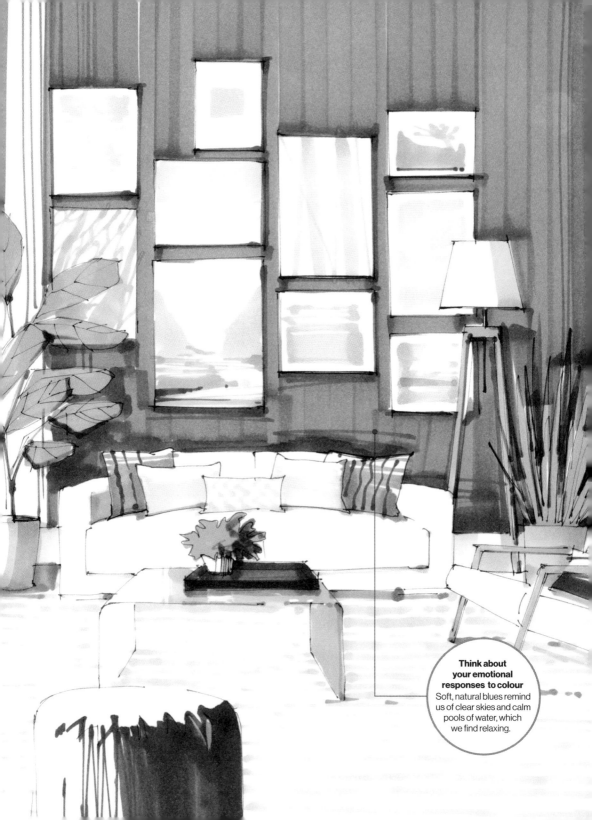

Think about your emotional responses to colour
Soft, natural blues remind us of clear skies and calm pools of water, which we find relaxing.

1 | Our perception of colour

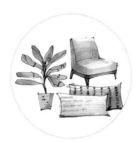

Colour in the home means much more than just painting the walls. We can also layer hues in furniture, flooring and fabrics, or artworks. Colours affect us physically and emotionally, but what causes this?

There are many colour theories, but for us the ecological valence theory proposed by psychologists Stephen E Palmer and Karen B Schloss best explains our colour preferences and responses. It suggests that we have different emotional responses to colours based on our associations with them; we react well to colours we experience positively. We tend to like colours that remind us of nature when it is thriving, as these signal health, life and safety.

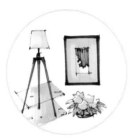

Imagine a room filled with:
• **soft, natural blues** – these bring to mind clear skies and cool, calm pools of water, so they help us feel relaxed.
• **shades of vibrant green** – these remind us of the energy and calm we experience in the middle of a natural meadow or forest.
• **yellows** – these remind us of warm summer sunshine, ripe crops and sunflowers; they are warming and welcoming and create an energized, social atmosphere.
• **purples and mauves** – these take us to the gentle light of the magic hours at dawn and dusk; they can also be mysterious, spiritual and meditative colours.
• **oranges and reds** – these remind us of ripe fruits and berries; the promise of nutrition can be energizing, exciting and stimulating.

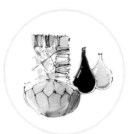

If you think about it, these natural elements were key to our survival not all that long ago. We have inherited these evolutionary preferences, so if we use them in our homes in the right ways and right places, they can support the way we want to feel at different times. Research into emotional responses to colour has found that pastel shades such as light green, lilac and blue were likely to make the participants feel calm, while brighter colours such as yellow, orange and pink made them feel more upbeat and excitable.
   If you want to introduce colour into your home, but feel daunted by the idea of making over your entire house, the following pages contain some top tips.

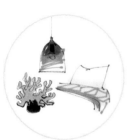

2 Plan your colour scheme

Colour is what we call a "natural analogue": something that references nature or natural systems without being the real thing.

Using natural colours that complement each other and follow a similar pattern to natural scenes will evoke a sense of a nature connection, even if there are no real elements of nature nearby. This will have a positive impact on the overall mood and feeling of a space, whether that's calming and relaxing or social and energizing.

First, decide how you want to feel in the space, then create a colour scheme around that. Try creating a mood board of nature scenes you'd like to draw inspiration from based on the desired atmosphere. Pinterest is great for keeping everything organized.

Getting the proportions right can determine whether colour feels too much or just right.

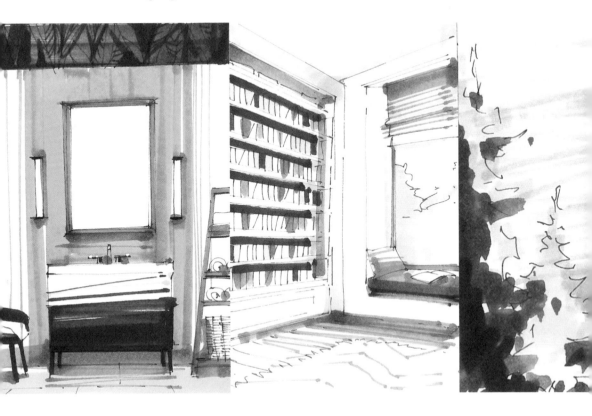

The trick is to not overwhelm the senses, but to use colours in your home in much the same proportions as you might find them in nature.

It's helpful to keep in mind that no colour is ever seen in isolation in a natural setting. If we look at a natural landscape, we notice how harmonious the many colours are. Woodlands have a variety of greens and browns, yet as a whole there is a sense of harmony. Even the pops of bright, contrasting colours of flowers on the forest floor don't seem out of place – they capture our attention in a positive way.

With that in mind, brightening up your home with colour doesn't have to mean painting all four walls the same shade; with a little creative thinking, your space can be bursting with life in no time. We want to strive for just the right

Use colours in your home in the same proportions as you might find them in nature.

balance of nature's proportions, harmony and contrasts so that we are comfortable but our senses are stimulated. After all, isn't this how we feel in nature?

When colour planning for a particular room, consider those natural layers and how you want to introduce them. Pull out colours from your mood board and place them around the room on walls, flooring, furniture, fixtures, fittings, and soft furnishings.

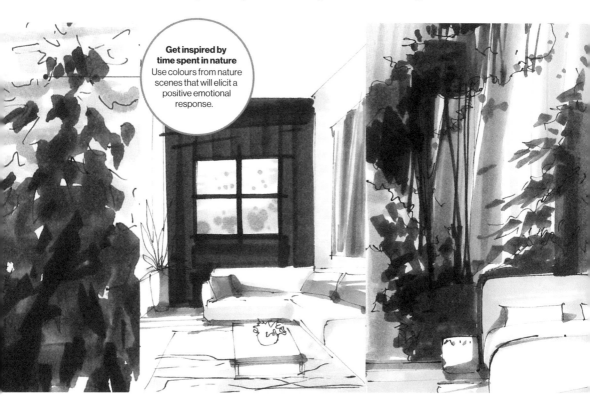

Get inspired by time spent in nature
Use colours from nature scenes that will elicit a positive emotional response.

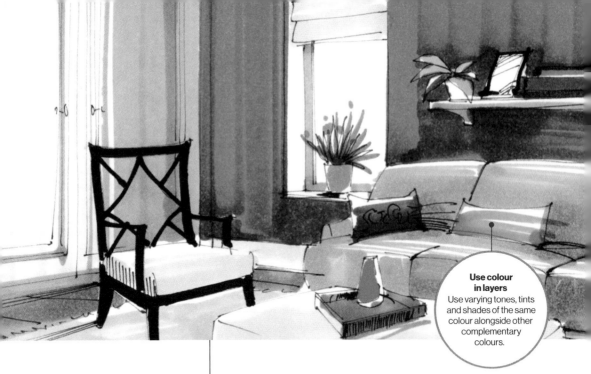

Use colour in layers
Use varying tones, tints and shades of the same colour alongside other complementary colours.

③ Create colour harmony

Your colour scheme and its layers need to be harmonious. In nature, colours aren't seen in isolation; the colours you choose for the walls provide the backdrop for the rest of the colour scheme (the furniture and furnishings).

There are two approaches to creating a harmonious colour scheme: using different shades, tones and tints of the same colour; or using adjacent colours on the colour wheel.

When it comes to paint, you'll need to consider the colour of the ceiling, skirting boards, doors and frames, windowsills and frames, shelves, cupboards or mantelpieces, as well as the walls. You can create subtle layers of the same colour by applying different tones, tints and shades of one colour. Starting with your main colour choice, you could add:

• **grey for varying tones**, to "tone down" the colour intensity. This is often considered more sophisticated; pure and bright colours are more playful. You can have very light tones or very dark tones, but none are vibrant.
• **white for varying tints**, to lighten the colour. Think of these as pastels; the colour is the same, but you have created a paler version. This will feel lighter, airier and softer.
• **black for varying shades**, or darker versions of your colour, from slightly darker to almost black; think of shadows to remind you. This will feel darker, moodier and have a deeper impact.

Alternatively, you could choose harmonious colours that sit next to each other on the

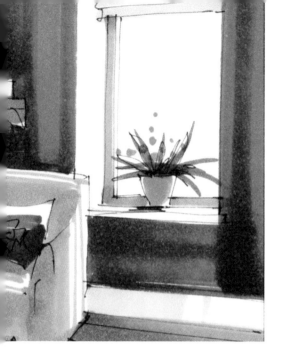

How light and colour interact

4

You'll need to work out whether your room is north or south facing before choosing your colour scheme.

In the northern hemisphere, north-facing rooms don't usually get warm, direct light, so warm tones will feel more welcoming. An east-facing room will get the morning light, but using warmer tones will ensure it's inviting for the rest of the day. A south-facing room can take cooler colours, because the light in here will often be warmer for the whole day.

All colours can have a warm or cool undertone. You can choose whatever colour you like – just opt for a warmer or a cooler undertone depending on the light in the space.

Colours will change depending on the time of day, and under natural or artificial light. Put a colour sample on a sheet of paper or a fabric swatch in place for 24 hours before deciding.

If you're still struggling to brighten up your space, light-reflective paints will bounce more light around the room. Using these near windows is a sure way to maximize this.

WARM TONES

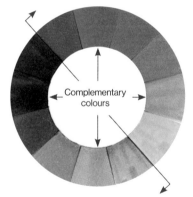

Complementary colours

COOL TONES

colour wheel. For example, if you have created layers with tints of green, you might want to add yellows or blues that will be more harmonious than, say, red. Your eye will make a very easy shift from one colour to the other, so this will have a calming effect. However, if you do want to create energy and contrast, consider adding pops of complementary colours.

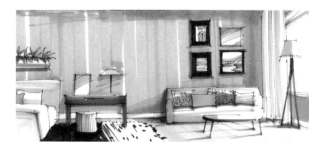

5 | Add pops of colour

A great way to introduce bolder colours without making the room feel small or oppressive is to use the idea of natural proportions.

Instead of painting solid blocks of colour on all the walls in a room, keep them to a feature wall or a half-height line of colour instead. Diagonal blocks can create a more dynamic feel by stimulating the eyes and mind to bring a sense of energy to a space.

Highlighting is also a great way to add colourful moments to your home without overwhelming a room. Examples of this are painting the back of your bookcase a vivid tone to make it pop, or painting the architrave of your door in an eye-catching tone to invite people in. Consider painting the wall or a section of wall behind a favourite mirror or wall hanging; if you're feeling brave, highlight it with an organic, fluid shape to really create a statement. Picking out special objects in this way allows us to introduce bursts of colour without it becoming over-stimulating.

You could even add a little playfulness to your staircase by painting the risers (the vertical panels). This technique works especially well in traditional

homes, as it brings together new and old by adding a contemporary flash of colour to characterful woodwork. Staircases are often seen as soon as we enter the home, so it's a great way to welcome people in and make them smile.

If you live in rented accommodation and can't paint anything, you can still create nature-inspired colour contrasts through your choice of furniture, soft furnishings and artwork. Choose complementary colours that are opposite each other on the colour wheel; the combination of warm and cool works very well. For example, in a blue or green room, consider bringing in small amounts of yellow or red as a contrast.

Why not make your own gallery of artworks above your sofa or in a hallway? This is a great solution for people who are renting, or love having flexibility and like to change things around regularly.

Consider investing in some statement furniture and furnishing pieces that add pops of colour. This could be a block-colour sofa, ombre-effect curtains, flamboyant cushions or two-toned throws and rugs. Layering different colours helps the space become visually rich and enticing.

Pick out special objects with accents of bold colour.

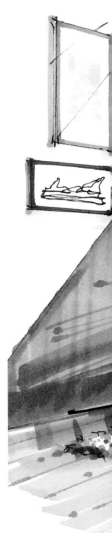

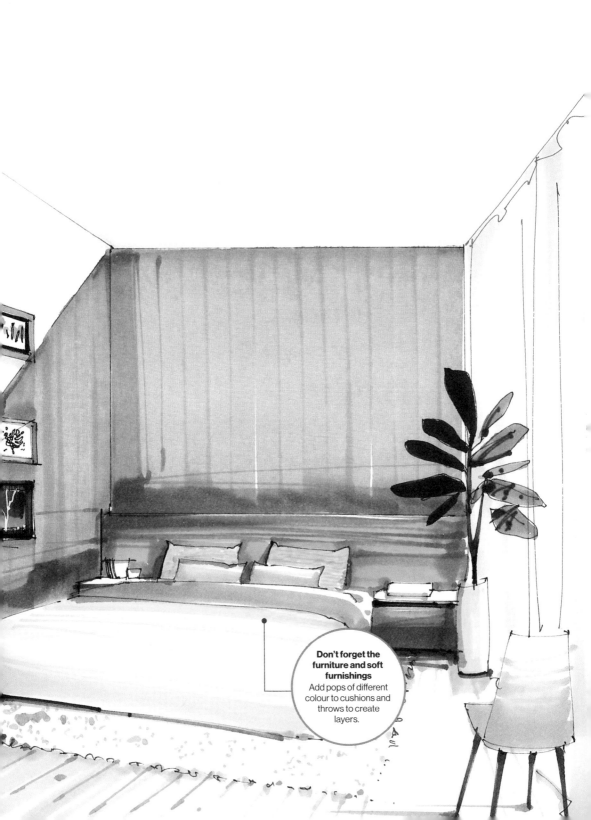

Don't forget the furniture and soft furnishings
Add pops of different colour to cushions and throws to create layers.

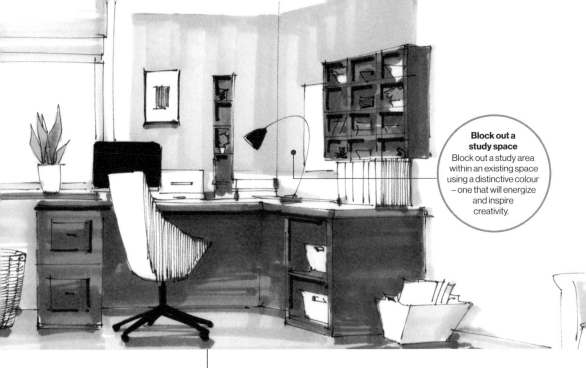

Block out a study space
Block out a study area within an existing space using a distinctive colour – one that will energize and inspire creativity.

 | # Zone using colour

If your home is open plan or has large rooms, consider zoning the different areas with accent colours.

Usually, areas are zoned where you want to step away from the main space into a place with a specific separate function. You could block out a study area in your living room with a distinctive colour, or highlight a reading nook with a mellow complementary hue.

Paint can be used in a graphic way, such as in bands of colour horizontally, vertically or diagonally that will immediately start to define spaces. This can be mixed with your choice of furniture, fabrics, and flooring colours.

This technique can enhance placemaking, especially if you live in a household with multiple people and activities going on. By forming subtle zones using colour, you can allocate different activities to different spaces. This will help keep everything in its place and reduce friction in the household.

By forming subtle zones using colour, you can allocate different activities to different spaces.

7 | Be careful with dark colours

It's easy to see why dark colours are a growing trend in home renovation. They're not only classic, but are often associated with sophistication, depth and mystery. However, if they aren't used carefully they can make your space feel oppressive and small. Here are some tips to help you tackle a dark palette confidently.

As in nature, darker spaces are associated with feelings of security and refuge, like being inside a cocoon or a cave. This is why darker tones work well for private, intimate spaces, such as a quiet reading nook, snug lounge or surrounding a cosy bed. Dark rooms can feel quite romantic, like a candle-lit dinner. When you use dark colours, you reduce reflected light bouncing around the room, meaning that light only emanates directly from the source, such as a window or light bulb.

Heavy use of dark colours can be dominating, so consider applying them in spaces you do not occupy for long periods of the day. An ideal location would be a hallway's half-height wall panelling, or a porch's floor tiling. These will make a bold statement upon entering the home, but remember that you don't have to paint every wall in the same colour. Instead, add layers and break up your spaces with splashes of dark colour.

When experimenting with darker tones, also carefully consider the lighting within each room. Brightly lit spaces can bring out rich, deep shades, but a low-lit space can make darker tones feel gloomy. If you have your heart set on dark colours, it may be worth saving them for the rooms with the biggest windows or the most lighting.

If you're anxious about low light levels, consider using a gloss paint on some surfaces to help bounce what light you do have around the room. It can create a stunning contrast as you move through the space. Be careful, though: gloss paint can also show up your wall's imperfections!

Finally, invigorate your dark palette by introducing pops of bright accent colour, such as a yellow radiator or vibrant red armchair, or with a thriving planting scheme – it will add an extra dimension and bring the room to life.

HOW TO CREATE DARK ACCENTS

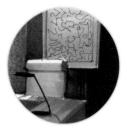

Darker colours work well in well-lit rooms, but can feel gloomy in poor natural light.

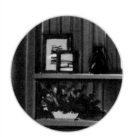

Bring dark surfaces to life with light-reflecting finishes and objects to create contrast.

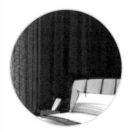

Dark tones work well surrounding a cosy bed for a cocoon-like feel.

Tune in to your fractal fluency

Imagine you are walking through a forest. What can you see? Branches are intertwined overhead, and their pattern is highlighted by the blue sky peeking through the gaps and casting shadows on the ground.

Perhaps you might notice patterns in the mixture of soil, undergrowth and fallen leaves, and how each inch of wood has its own unique markings.

Now take a leaf in your hand. As you look closely, you see the pattern of its veins repeating itself over and over again at increasingly smaller scales. These organic repeating patterns are derived from dynamic processes in nature, and are known as biophilic fractals. Others include the way a river has shaped the land, how cracked dirt can become canyons if you look closely enough. Fractal patterns can be found in mountains, sand dunes, coral reefs, beehives, snowflakes, flowers, pinecones, shells, pebbles... the list is endless.

Our ancestors would have used these patterns to identify and navigate landscapes, and we have inherited a "fractal fluency", or a preference for natural fractal patterns ingrained in our very being. In fact, research has found that viewing fractals can reduce stress by 60%, and it can also have a restorative effect.

If natural patterns can enhance overall health and wellbeing, why not consider adding some into your home? Next, we'll explore how and where this can be done.

Types of fractal
Biophilic fractals are more appealing to us than manmade "exact fractals" because they are less precise and have occurred naturally.

Fractal fluency is a preference for natural fractal patterns ingrained in our very being.

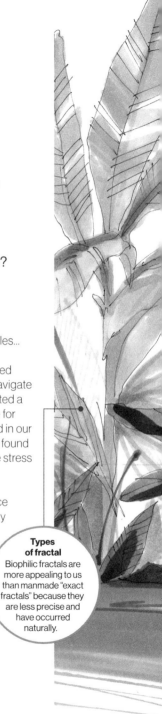

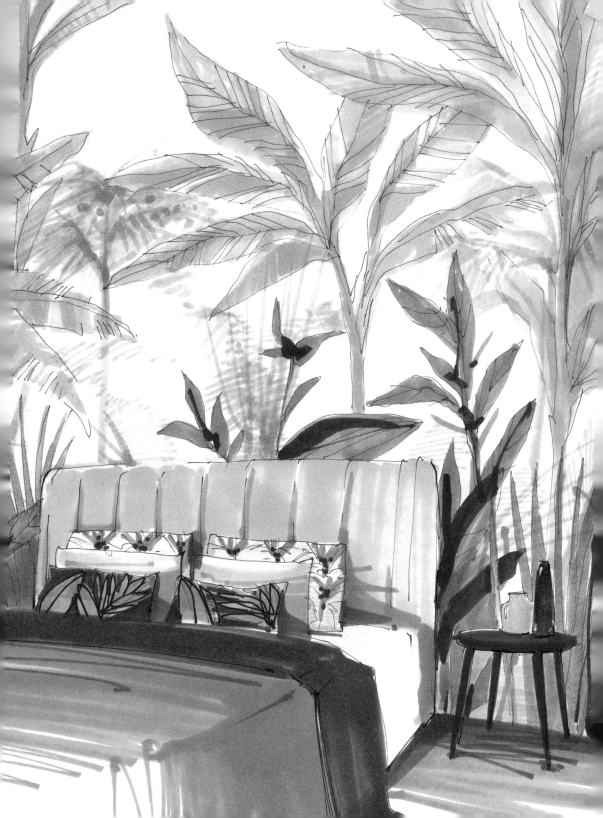

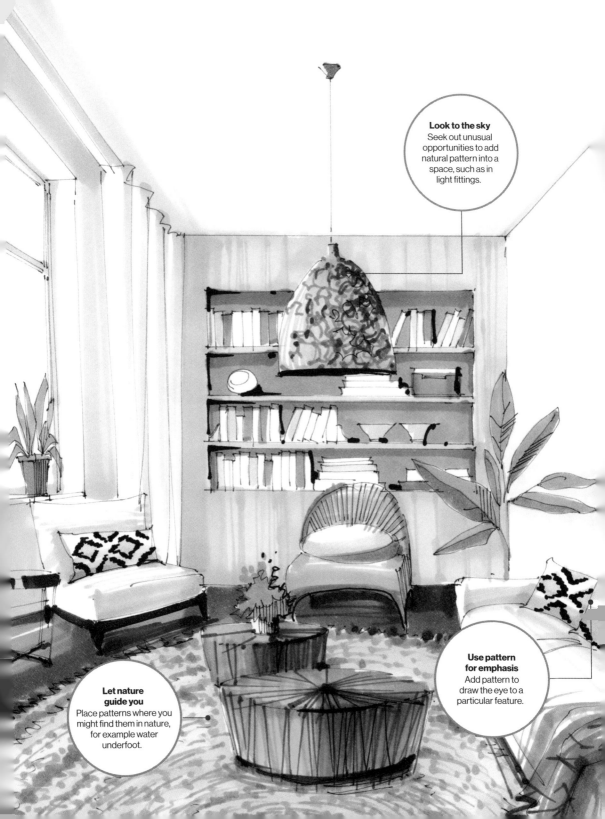

Look to the sky
Seek out unusual opportunities to add natural pattern into a space, such as in light fittings.

Use pattern for emphasis
Add pattern to draw the eye to a particular feature.

Let nature guide you
Place patterns where you might find them in nature, for example water underfoot.

Use pattern in the right places

Unlike other mammals, humans have an expanded cerebral cortex (the outer layer of the brain), which means we have more synapses and neurons, the cells and connections that help the brain process information. This has enabled us to develop superior pattern processing. In fact, more than half of cortex function is dedicated to processing visual information, including patterns, rather than other sensory stimuli like sounds and touch.

Visual patterns found in nature can be introduced into our homes in all sorts of ways, from lampshades with cut-outs that cast shadows around the room, to illustrated or graphic wallpapers (for example, with forest scenes on them). Patterns can even be introduced in the placement of artwork, stencilled images or pictures on a wall, for example if they are hung in a scattered positioning or a spiral formation.

Observing patterns in nature was an important part of how our ancestors made sense of environments. It follows, then, that indoors they should be placed where we would find them in the natural world.

Let's look at the leaf pattern again as an example. In nature, you might find fallen leaves on the ground or growing on high and low plants, branches and bushes, so leaf-like patterns can work just about anywhere: on rugs to mimic the forest floor, or on throws, cushions, wallpaper and curtains, all at the height of different types of foliage. Flooring or rugs that have patterns like water, soil, grass, rocks, or sand would make sense underfoot, as this is where you find them in nature; but flooring that mimics the sky could be disorientating.

Sticking to the natural hierarchy and placement of pattern can create more harmonious spaces that have complexity and order at the same time. We can make use of rich sensory information while ensuring we do not become overwhelmed by working with nature's spatial hierarchy and proportions. This offers reassurance that everything is in its natural place, which helps you and others to feel comfortable in your home.

Biomorphic forms are man-made objects in a shape reminiscent of something that exists in nature; for example a pebble-shaped footstool or beehive-shaped shelving. They are another great way of introducing nature-inspired patterns into the home.

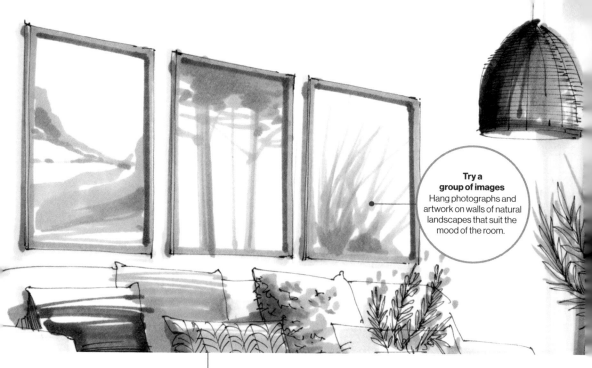

Try a group of images
Hang photographs and artwork on walls of natural landscapes that suit the mood of the room.

10 | Bring in natural patterns with images

Displaying natural patterns is great for health and wellbeing. Studies have found that a vast majority of people have a preference for artworks containing biophilic fractal patterns over other types of pattern.

Projections of fractal patterns onto floors and walls have been found to enhance visual interest and mood more than non-fractal patterns. Importantly, hospital patients rate artworks depicting elements of nature such as greenery, flowers, trees and water positively, but they experience increased anxiety if the artwork is abstract.

There are many ways to bring images of nature into your home. You can, of course, display photographs of natural scenes on your shelves and walls, drawing from your own experiences. Alternatively, you could choose artworks such as prints, drawings or paintings. These might be of vast landscapes or close-ups of natural objects that feel more abstract, but both contain those all-important biophilic fractals.

Before you hang your image or artwork, think about how it makes you feel. A photo of sunlight gently shining through a forest canopy may be suited to relaxing, calm spaces, but a lively seascape might better suit a room where you want to feel invigorated.

Finally, consider the scale and how many nature images you want to display in each room. You might want one big focal point for the room or a cluster of smaller images that draw you in and feature different types of subtle biophilic pattern.

11 | Zone using pattern

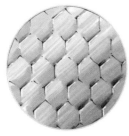

We tend to feel more comfortable when we know what a space is for. The home is no exception; it is made up of smaller spaces, each of which fulfils a different purpose. Patterns can be used to create zones within spaces so that each one has a slightly different look or feel.

Consider how you can use visual pattern to define a space for its purpose and activity, whether that's calming, relaxing, restorative or energizing.

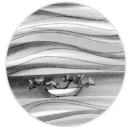

• In the **bathroom**, you might want to use rippled or soft undulating patterns to remind yourself of the calmness of water; think water surface, sand or shell patterns.
• In the **living room**, leafy patterns and forest-inspired shapes and patterns can be relaxing and restorative.
• **Retreats** or **quiet spaces** such as bedrooms or home offices might benefit from images of sheltered or secluded natural spaces, for example cave-like patterns.
• By contrast, **lively spaces** may suit patterns of more dynamic natural systems, such as waterfalls and rivers.

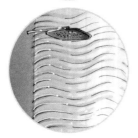

Remember that there is a balance to strive for here. Subtlety is key, so that the patterns don't dominate the space and overwhelm you. Also keep in mind that there are no straight lines in nature, so hard edges can appear harsh. Now, why not get out in nature, observe the patterns and be inspired by the natural world?

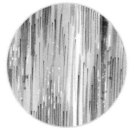

Subtlety is key, so that the patterns don't dominate the space and overwhelm you.

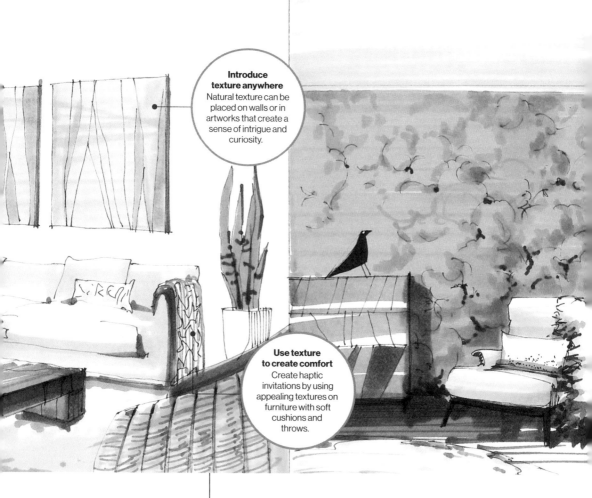

Introduce texture anywhere
Natural texture can be placed on walls or in artworks that create a sense of intrigue and curiosity.

Use texture to create comfort
Create haptic invitations by using appealing textures on furniture with soft cushions and throws.

12 Feel the benefit of natural textures

We've seen how colour and pattern can help us forge beneficial connections with nature, but now let's take a look at texture. How can we harness different textures in the home to maximize our wellbeing?

During much of our evolution, we humans would have had daily physical contact with the feathers, fur or scales of animals; water, rocks, pebbles and sand; and all the different kinds of grasses and plants you can imagine.

Even today, our wellbeing is negatively impacted if spaces are lacking in texture. We can experience tactile deprivation and "touch hunger". Textures are something we both feel and see, and having an array of textures in a

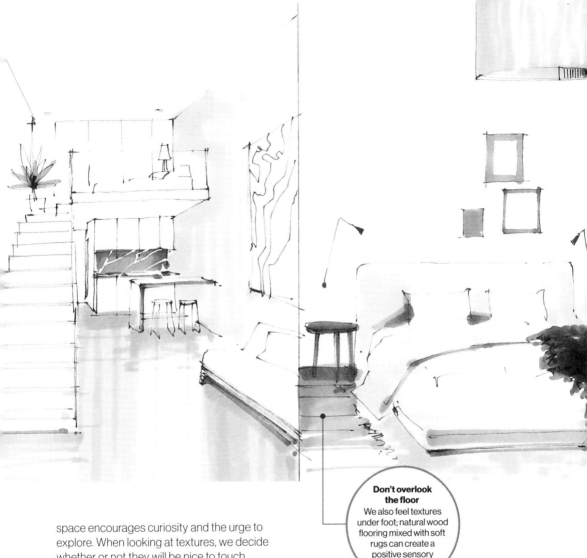

**Don't overlook
the floor**
We also feel textures
under foot; natural wood
flooring mixed with soft
rugs can create a
positive sensory
journey.

space encourages curiosity and the urge to explore. When looking at textures, we decide whether or not they will be nice to touch, immediately calculating their "touch-ability".

If a texture looks inviting, we take this as a "haptic invitation" (an appeal to our sense of touch to have a positive tactile experience). These experiences can create a sense of belonging, and we feel more comfortable if we are surrounded by appealing textures.

We need to consider how textures look as well as how they feel, because we experience them through both senses. We might keep the grain on wood, or bring in other natural materials that both look and feel inviting.

If a texture looks inviting, we take this as a "haptic invitation" – an appeal to our sense of touch to have a positive tactile experience.

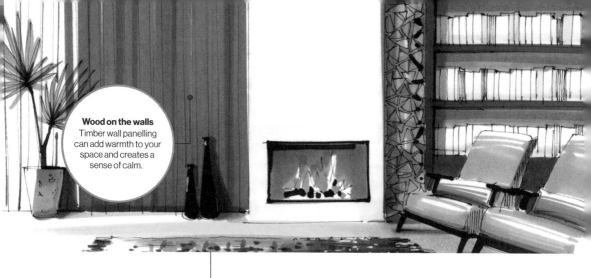

Wood on the walls
Timber wall panelling can add warmth to your space and creates a sense of calm.

13 | Use wood

Humans have used trees to build homes since civilization began. In this sense, we have a deeply rooted, inherent connection to timber because it has provided us with shelter and warmth. In fact, it seems that as our lives have become fast-paced and digitalized, this relationship has deepened; many of us seek out natural materials for our homes, such as timber.

Every piece of wood has a distinctive character that no manmade product can replicate: it is unique and one of a kind. A beautiful hardwood floor or oak kitchen worktop has an authentic, warm, reliable quality, but the use of timber in our homes goes way beyond visual attraction. The presence of wood has clear positive effects: using it on walls, floors and ceilings has been found to reduce blood pressure and increase comfort. Research into the effects of exposure to wood on wellbeing revealed even more positive outcomes. Optimism about the future increased by 17%, confidence levels increased by 19% and stress levels plummeted by 23%. What's not to like about that?

Using timber is a win-win for us and the planet. It is a hardwearing, renewable and beautiful building material, and trees take in carbon dioxide through photosynthesis as they grow. When they are cut down, the carbon is locked in, not released, so using responsibly sourced timber instead of carbon-intensive materials like steel can reduce your carbon footprint.

Consider bringing warmth into your space with timber wall panelling, or expose floorboards or wooden beams to add character and charm. Keep the natural grain for added visual and tactile benefits.

Other ways of using wood in the home include: timber handles and handrails, driftwood ornaments, or coffee tables and shelves with waney edges (this is when one edge is left with the natural shape of the tree; sometimes the bark is left on too).

14 | Connect with nature through materials

Creating a material connection with nature is a fundamental part of the biophilic design approach. It is defined as bringing materials, surfaces and textures that are found in nature into the built environment. Ideally, these will have gone through minimal processing so that they reflect the local geology or ecology, to create a sense of place.

In the home, it is important to include a variety of textures, just as you would find in nature, in order to create some of those "haptic invitations", or prompts to have a pleasurable tactile experience.

You might take inspiration from the textures of your immediate natural environment to enhance a sense of belonging, as this can be beneficial to your wellbeing. Alternatively, source materials and textures that transport you back to fond memories of time spent in nature to create your own sense of place.

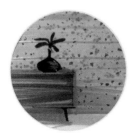

Cork and leather

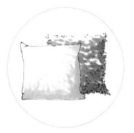

Soft woven fabrics on cushions

Other ways to create material connections in your home include:

Sheepskin rugs or throws

Varied textural fabrics

Cool marble surfaces

Clay or ceramic furnishings and fittings

Use of bark

Rattan seating

Moss walls (made from preserved moss, these come as panels and don't need light, water or soil)

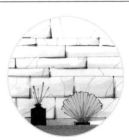

Using stones, pebbles and shells as ornaments

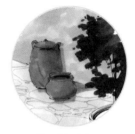

Unpolished stone surfaces

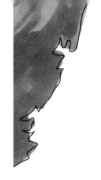

15 Create mindful moments

We can create sensory journeys in the home that promote mindfulness by using different types of flooring and wall coverings, or hard or soft furnishings. Textural contrasts disrupt the sensory habituation of monotonous surfaces, creating rich, varied experiences that keep you present in the moment.

When we feel different textures underfoot we are pulled into the moment as we notice the change in surface texture, hardness and temperature. We have an instinctive vestibular (balance) response to texture, just as we have a visual and haptic response. In nature, we have to adjust our motion and balance in response to what we are stepping on. Think about how you run across hot sand or hobble over a pebbly beach. What about the sensation you notice when you stand for the first time on something cold, rough or soft? For a moment you focus on how it feels, creating an awareness of the present moment and your surroundings, in contrast to moving through a space on autopilot, as we so often do.

Different materials and surfaces in nature have different sensory qualities, so these effects can be recreated in any space of the home. Think about when you wake up in the morning and imagine a sensory journey from your bed to your bathroom; as you swing your legs out of bed your feet touch a soft wool rug. Next, you walk across the warm wooden floor and step onto cool bathroom tiles before immersing yourself in an invigorating hot shower.

Things as simple as these moments of increased sensory awareness can help pull us out of sleep and set us up for the day ahead.

One final consideration is which materials sit well next to each other. We have discussed the haptic invitation of textural contrast, but textures should also be harmonious. For example, on your sofa you might have a sheepskin throw next to a yarn cushion, which is slightly firmer in texture. Having a good balance of textures is key to reaping the benefits.

Further, a wooden countertop is warmer than, say, a marble one, so these feel different to the touch. Resting your arms on a marble kitchen counter might be nice and cooling in summer, but a timber dining table would be cosier in the winter months. Try to think about the material qualities your home offers and how you might use these to elicit a different response to the space. Cool, hard surfaces are energizing and active, and warm, soft surfaces are calming and restorative. Creating a sensory textural journey through your home is an exciting way to design a space that subtly soothes and refreshes your mental and physical states. Why not give it a go?

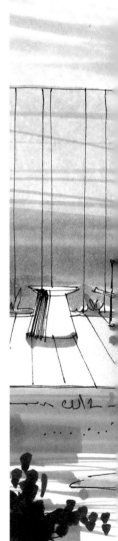

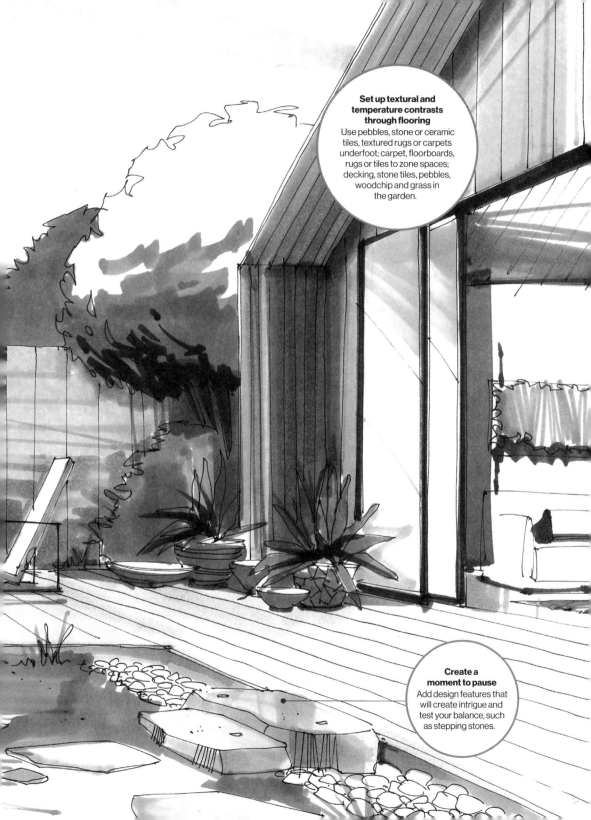

Set up textural and temperature contrasts through flooring
Use pebbles, stone or ceramic tiles, textured rugs or carpets underfoot; carpet, floorboards, rugs or tiles to zone spaces; decking, stone tiles, pebbles, woodchip and grass in the garden.

Create a moment to pause
Add design features that will create intrigue and test your balance, such as stepping stones.

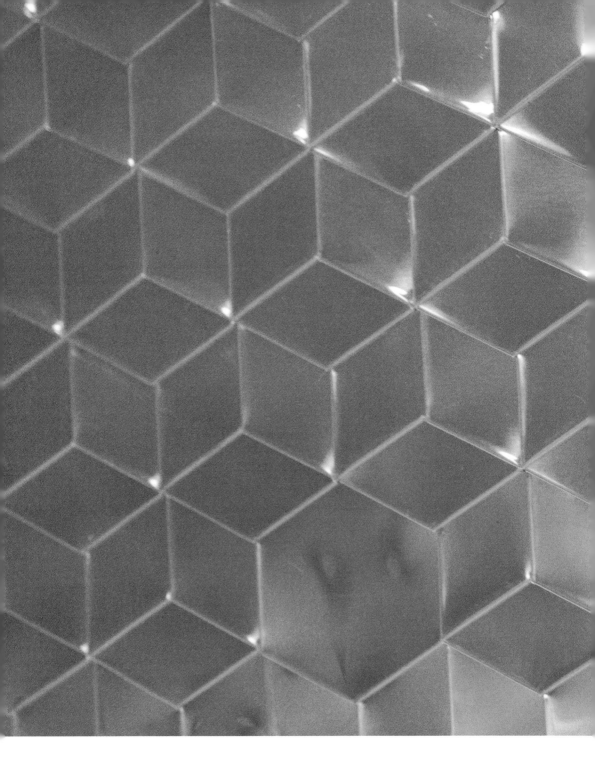

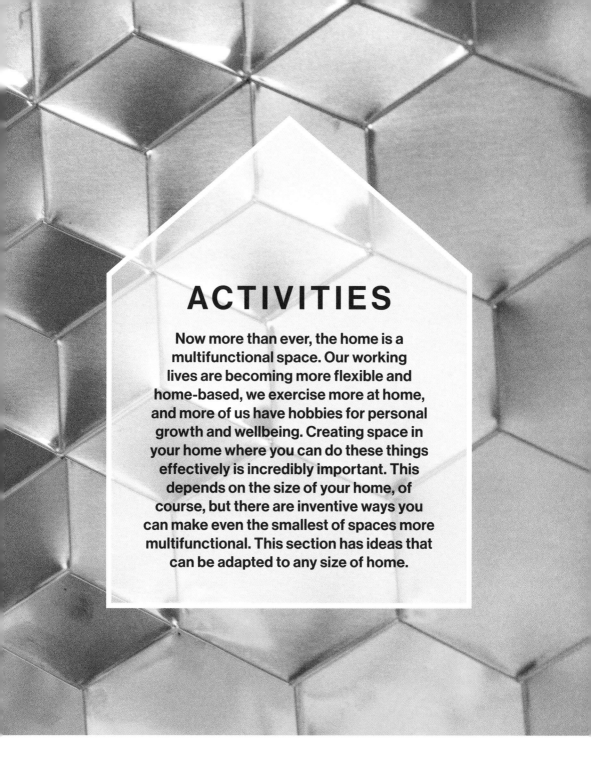

ACTIVITIES

Now more than ever, the home is a multifunctional space. Our working lives are becoming more flexible and home-based, we exercise more at home, and more of us have hobbies for personal growth and wellbeing. Creating space in your home where you can do these things effectively is incredibly important. This depends on the size of your home, of course, but there are inventive ways you can make even the smallest of spaces more multifunctional. This section has ideas that can be adapted to any size of home.

16 | Create a workspace

Even before the COVID-19 pandemic, surveys revealed that nearly half of all Britons sometimes worked from home, but only 11% of those had a designated space to work, and 1 in 10 people admitted that they often work from their sofa! Clearly, this is not much good for our health and wellbeing, especially since working from home is now more common than before.

When designing a much-needed home office, first and foremost we need to consider its location. This can have a huge impact on our ability to work. Many people won't have much choice in this, but somewhere as acoustically and visually separated from the rest of the house as possible is ideal. This separation is the best approach to aiding productive and focused work. If possible, don't make it your bedroom; the bedroom is your place to relax and feel restored, not somewhere you want to be reminded of work.

Having your own room for an office would, of course, be the easiest way to do this. Even if you don't have a spare room to dedicate solely to this, you might have a room big enough to section part off with a planted partition to work behind. This can be as simple as open shelving with potted plants to add a feeling of separation; it signals that you don't want to be disturbed, and allows you to take calls or video meetings without feeling overlooked.

Once you've found your spot, think about the layout. Position your desk under a window, if possible, as this will maximize your exposure to natural light and can aid focus, especially if you have a view out onto greenery. Studies have shown that a view of nature can increase work performance by 10–25%. Looking out of your window and being able to connect with natural systems, such as noticing the seasons and weather patterns as they change, enhances wellbeing.

Keeping this space organized is also important. We can all relate to the stressful experience of rifling through a box of papers to find that one receipt from last month. Having a well-organized space with proper storage helps us live and work more efficiently, with less hassle, which means we have a clear head to work productively.

Enhance wellbeing
Position your desk under or near a window to maximize exposure to natural light and notice seasonal changes outside.

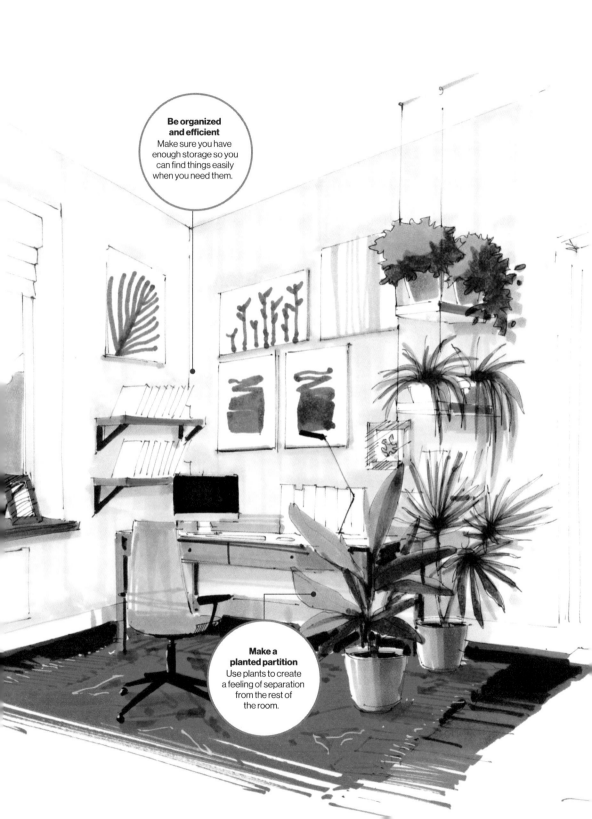

Be organized and efficient
Make sure you have enough storage so you can find things easily when you need them.

Make a planted partition
Use plants to create a feeling of separation from the rest of the room.

17 | The ergonomics of working from home

If you spend a lot of time sitting at a computer, it's vital that your home office furniture is set up correctly to support your spine and protect your physical health. This minimizes discomfort and boosts your productivity. Did you just sit up straighter? Here's how to set up an ergonomic home office.

Position your screen at eye level and make sure it's an arm's length away from you. This will help prevent you from slouching over and straining your neck, and will encourage you to sit up straight. Check that your eyebrows are in line with the top of your screen, then stretch out your arms and check that your fingers can just touch the screen in front of you.

Additionally, make sure your back is adequately supported. Investing in an

ergonomic office chair that allows you to adjust the backrest position to meet the small of your lower back can reduce back strain. If your chair has arm rests, ensure you adjust these to where your elbow naturally hangs, so your shoulders stay relaxed and not tense.

You could also consider investing in a sit/stand desk. Standing desks have been linked to many physiological and psychological health benefits, including improved moods

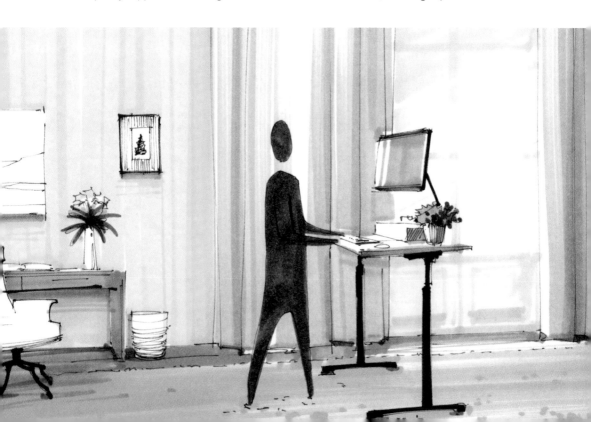

and stress reduction. One study showed that 87% of people using standing desks daily reported increased energy levels throughout the day, and moods went back to their original levels once the standing desk was removed.

An armchair with a side table and lamp will provide a space away from your screen for tasks that don't need a desk (and you won't leave your office to read on the sofa). Having a choice of seating and lighting options can add a feeling of control within a space, which has been shown to improve wellbeing.

Finally, don't forget how important it is to take regular breaks and stretch; short, frequent breaks are proven to be more effective than long, less frequent ones. For example, taking a 5–10 minute break once an hour is more effective than, say, taking 20 minutes every two hours. This will minimize prolonged periods of sitting in the same position.

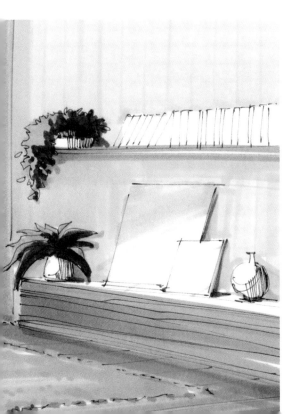

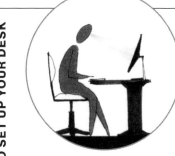

Take note of the angle of your head, back and the way that your feet touch the ground.

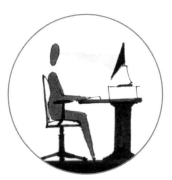

Position your screen at eye level, an arm's length away from you, and make sure your chair allows you to put your feet flat on the ground.

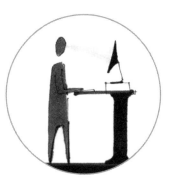

Consider investing in a sit/stand desk to enhance opportunities for better posture and ergonomics.

18 | Reduce distractions when home working

Working from home has its pros and cons. At least we don't have the background chatter of colleagues on calls or in meetings, or interruptions for conversations – but we do have a different set of distractions.

We might have housemates, partners, kids, pets, cleaners, the temptation to sort out the kitchen cupboards, or other elements of our domestic lives impinging on our ability to focus. We can also be distracted by design elements such as poor lighting and inadequate desk space.

We also have digital distractions to contend with. With mobile digital technology, we can have constant contact with friends and family on social media and direct messaging. We find these notifications extremely difficult to ignore; the average phone user touches their phone 2,617 times a day. In fact, just having a mobile phone on your desk can slow down your performance. Distractions like these are not only bad for our productivity, but also our mental and physical wellbeing.

First of all, try turning off your social media and instant messaging notifications when you're trying to focus. You could put your phone on flight mode to get your head down for a "power hour".

Secondly, try to have visual and acoustic separation from the rest of the house. If that's not working for you, try adding subtle natural background noise from an internal water feature; incorporating water into a workspace can enhance relaxation, positive emotions and concentration. If you like the idea of background noise but not a water feature, you can play natural sounds such as birdsong or gently running water through speakers in your workspace. Background noise will help mask any unwanted sounds and help you stay on task.

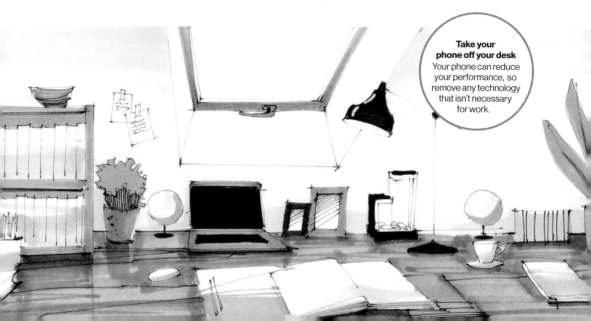

Take your phone off your desk
Your phone can reduce your performance, so remove any technology that isn't necessary for work.

How to restore focus

When our attention is pulled away from the task at hand, or we begin to feel tired from too much concentration, there are things we can do to refocus.

Non-rhythmic sensory stimuli (NRSS) are calming, gentle, non-threatening movements found in nature, such as ripples on a pool of water, grass swaying or leaves moving in a breeze, which can aid psychological restoration and reduce eyestrain from computers. The movement catches our eye every so often and allows us a moment of effortless attention on something in the distance. This is particularly beneficial if we refocus our vision every 20 minutes, for 20 seconds, on something 20 feet away (this is known as the 20x20x20 rule).

Adding some greenery to your workspace can help with this. Try placing a leafy plant next to an open window for gentle movement in a breeze. Aside from providing NRSS, plants can filter the air, remove toxins, introduce natural scent (rosemary is good for focus and memory) and generally improve productivity. Some plants increase the air's humidity, which reduces eye, nose and throat irritation.

One study found that the addition of plants visible from a workspace led to a 10% improvement in task performance, a 65% improvement in reported health and a 78% improvement in reported happiness – so plants help not only with focus and concentration but also physical and mental health and wellbeing.

Non-rhythmic sensory stimuli (NRSS) are calming, gentle, non-threatening movements found in nature.

NON-RHYTHMIC SENSORY STIMULI

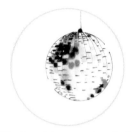

A kinetic sculpture or moving reflective object (think disco ball or mobile) can create glints of light that pull our attention.

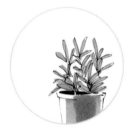

Fragrant plants such as rosemary introduce natural scenting and enhance focus and memory.

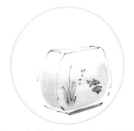

The gentle ripple of water in a fish tank is a great example of NRSS and allows for soft fascination.

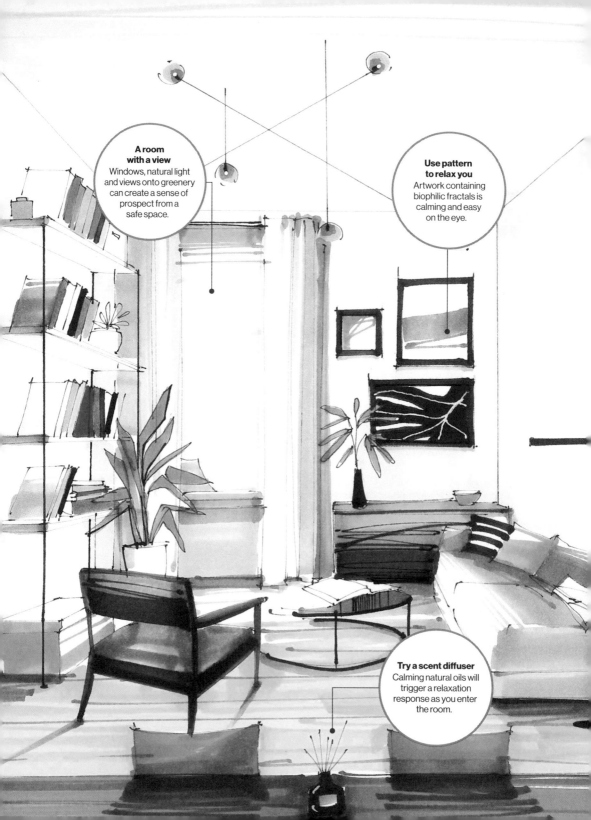

**A room
with a view**
Windows, natural light
and views onto greenery
can create a sense of
prospect from a
safe space.

**Use pattern
to relax you**
Artwork containing
biophilic fractals is
calming and easy
on the eye.

Try a scent diffuser
Calming natural oils will
trigger a relaxation
response as you enter
the room.

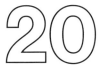

20 | Create a private space

Everyone needs their private space. It's so important to take a step back and recuperate without interruption in a space where we feel safe and calm.

We usually feel this sense of refuge in places that are sheltered, covered from behind, and have a view – out of a window, or at least across the rest of the room. In ancient times we might have sheltered in a cave or rested up against a tree. The "prospect-refuge" theory states that we have an inborn desire for prospect (in the sense of an extended view on to something) so that we can observe our surroundings without being seen by others. It is in these situations that we feel most relaxed.

How do we create this in the home? It could be as simple as having a high-backed chair in the corner of a room, a window seat to perch at or a small reading nook tucked away in a calm area. If you have the space, you could even create your own "wellness room".

> **The "prospect refuge" theory states that we have an inborn desire for a view, so that we can observe our surroundings.**

Imagine a room you could go to for some time out, to switch off or to meditate. What would you find in there? In addition to the seating options already suggested, here are some other things we know to be beneficial.

- **Windows and natural light**
- **Views out onto greenery** (or add some window planters)
- **A timber-cladded wall** or **timber furniture** to make the space feel warm and rich
- **Artwork** containing biophilic fractals (see page 24)
- **An immersive planting scheme** where you can sit among the foliage
- **Soft, natural fabrics** and textures
- **Adjustable lighting** (salt lamps give off a lovely warm glow)
- **A scent diffuser**
- **Carefully considered colours** to suit the mood you wish to create
- **A lock on the door** if you need it
- **Your favourite things that help you relax:** perhaps a TV, a selection of things to read, or whatever you need in order to feel as though you've given yourself a break.

21 | Make space for hobbies

With more activities squeezed into the home than ever before as our work and home lives collide, in a bid for some off-screen down time, people are turning to hobbies that they find calming, therapeutic and engaging. Working on a project for yourself will give you a sense of accomplishment and satisfaction.

If you have a hobby that you do at home – such as DIY, sewing, painting, jewellery making, embroidery, knitting, writing, music – try to create a space where you go to do it, or at least somewhere to store your equipment, so that it doesn't take over your house. This will reduce stress from clutter, and also make it possible to squeeze in your hobby time; we all know how tricky this can be, so make the most of this valuable time by being ready to get going whenever you find a moment.

Consider being fun with your design in these creative spaces. You could use design features to stimulate the senses and inspire you, for example:

• **incorporating a range of textures** on surfaces and furnishings for interest and variation.

• **using pops of colour** that enliven you, such as yellows and reds.
• **artwork on the walls**, of your favourite bands or your favourite paintings, or photos that inspire you.
• **a showcase** for whatever you've made, whether that's sculptures, wall hangings, pots, throws or books.

If the main aim of your hobby is to relax you, you might like a comfortable armchair with soft furnishings or a neutral, clutter-free area to clear your mind. You can create whatever atmosphere you want, whether that's fun or relaxing, by thinking about the design. Remember: this is a space for you!

Make proper storage space
Store your hobby equipment to reduce clutter, stay organized and allow you to find everything you need.

Be fun with your design in creative spaces, using design features to stimulate the senses and inspire you.

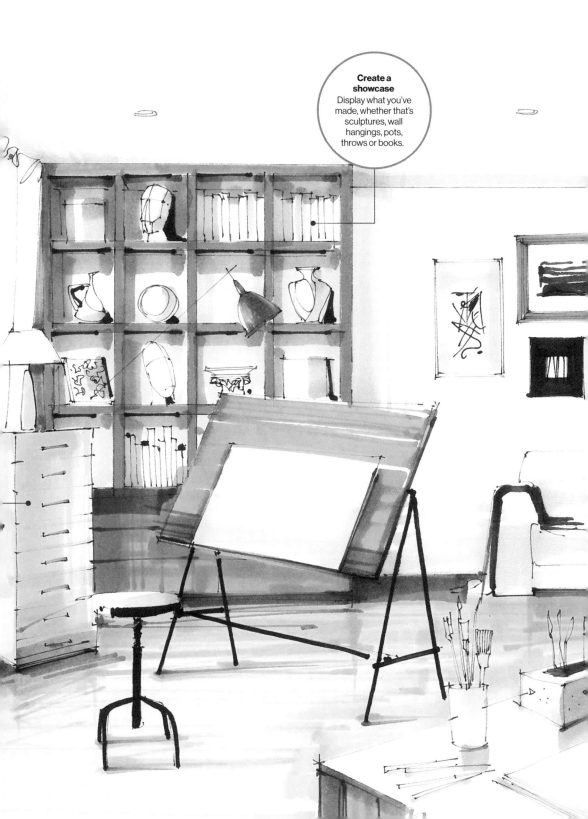

Create a showcase
Display what you've made, whether that's sculptures, wall hangings, pots, throws or books.

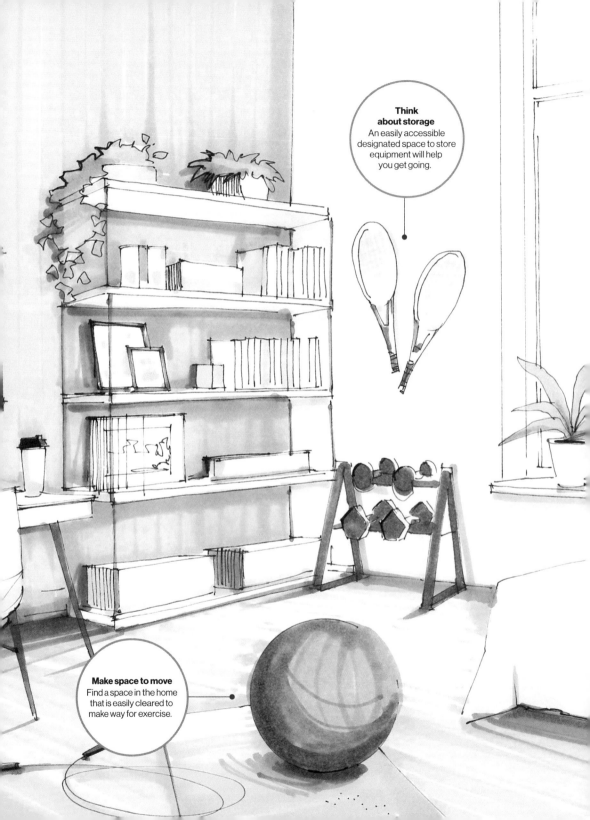

Think about storage
An easily accessible designated space to store equipment will help you get going.

Make space to move
Find a space in the home that is easily cleared to make way for exercise.

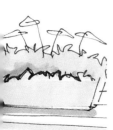

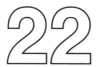

22 | Designate space for exercise

The COVID-19 pandemic highlighted what an important part of our lives exercise is. Only being allowed out once a day and a sudden shift to working from home made it hard to get in the daily steps that previously had just been part of the normal day. But we all know how beneficial exercise can be, from weight control and improved mental and physical health, to healthier gut biomes.

Try to make sure, then, that you have somewhere in your house where you can do a workout, whether that's yoga, core-strength exercises or an online class. If you know you have the space, it's harder to make an excuse as to why you can't fit a bit of movement into your morning, lunch break or after work.

Where should this space be? Many people work out in their living room,

and here, furniture that can be easily rearranged is key, such as a lightweight coffee table you can slide out of the way to give yourself enough space. If you have a spare room, consider a fold-away bed to free up the floor space when you don't have guests.

Having an easily accessible designated place to store any equipment is crucial for motivating you to exercise; if your weights, mat, resistance bands and foam roller are all strewn across different corners of the house, it's going to seem like more of an effort to get set up. If everything you need is stored in one place, you won't spend as long getting ready as you do on the workout!

If you know you have the space, it's harder to find an excuse not to exercise.

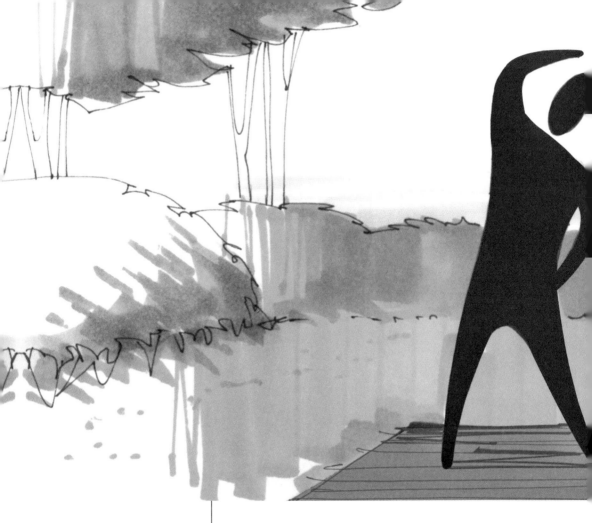

23 | **Exercise in garden spaces**

Mindfully immersing yourself in nature is a Japanese practice known as forest bathing, or *shinrin-yoku*.

The Japanese government values this practice so highly that it has spent over US$4 million researching the benefits of *shinrin-yoku* since 2003, and the results have been nothing but positive. Time spent in nature helps us to be more mindful, and to recuperate from

strenuous physical and mental activity faster.

At home, getting outside into the garden to exercise will create a more mindful and beneficial experience. Think about it: you are completing a series of exercises, and while you might initially have been more

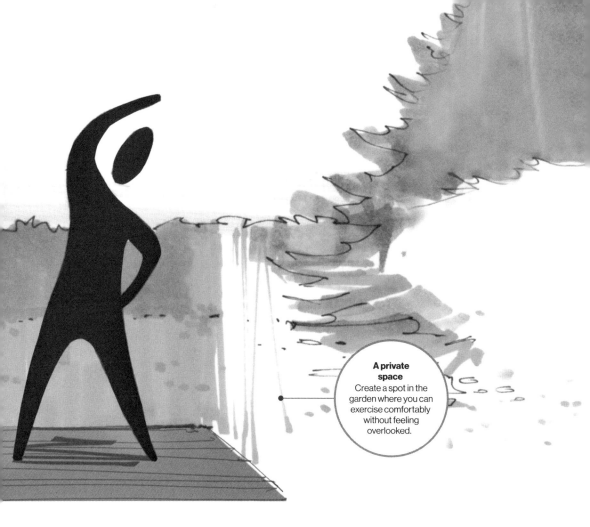

A private space
Create a spot in the garden where you can exercise comfortably without feeling overlooked.

comfortable in your living room, you soon warm up, and the cooler, fresh air is welcome. As you pause to rest, you might notice the quality of light, the weather and what it might bring that day, the subtle changes of shifting seasons, the sounds and movement of foliage in a breeze or the birds in the sky. You appreciate the natural sensory input and are aware of its richness and diversity.

Of course, you need to have a garden to do this. If you do, consider how you might design it to make exercise as easy and as comfortable as possible. Create a space that is large enough to move around in, flat, stable,

Time spent in nature helps us be more mindful, and recuperate from strenuous physical and mental activity faster.

non-slip and easy to clean. If feeling overlooked by neighbours puts you off exercising in the garden, add some privacy by screening your workout area off with trellis, bamboo slats or tall planting.

24 | Make sure you're ready to go out

While exercising at home is convenient and quick, research has shown that exercising in nature further afield can lower heart rates and result in greater heart rate variability. Here's how you can be ready to get outside.

Exercising in nature also goes hand in hand with reduced anxiety and elevated mood. In recent years, UK doctors have even been prescribing getting out and spending time in nature as a way of improving mental health.

How can our home help us get outside? Having everything ready to grab and go can stop you making excuses about getting out and exercising. Too hot out? You've got your water bottle, shorts and vest. Too cold? You've got long leggings and a jumper you can jog in.

Raining? That's why you bought a breathable rain jacket for exercising when it's wet. Have a place in your wardrobe specifically for your exercise clothing and a box by your front door for walking boots, wellies and trainers to remind you to get out.

If you cycle, storing your bike can be a hassle. Ideally, you'll have some kind of easily accessible storage outside the front of your home. If not, consider mounting your bike on an inside or outside wall so it doesn't take up

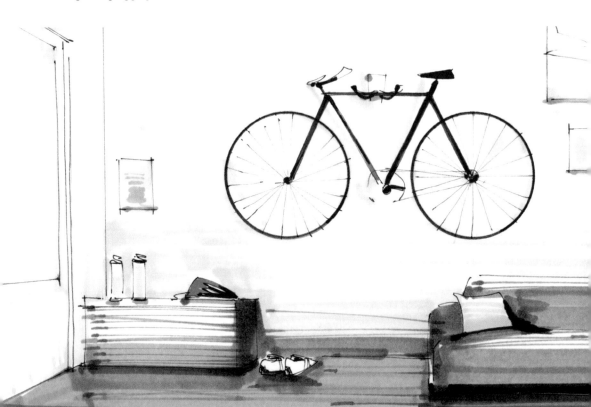

precious floorspace or block the hallway. If you notice your tyres are looking a bit flat, try not to leave it until next time you want to go out – pump them up as soon as you notice, so your bike is ready to go next time. Your future self will thank you!

If you're not sure where to start, or you don't have the confidence to exercise outdoors, consider getting involved in activities such as the NHS's Couch to 5K challenge, GoodGym (a community of runners who combine exercise with helping out in the local community), or Parkrun (regular Saturday morning 5km runs in more than 2,000 locations). These, and schemes like them, can provide a helpful way to motivate yourself to leave the house. They will also increase your sense of connection to the people and places in your local area. Exercising with others in green spaces will do you the world of good.

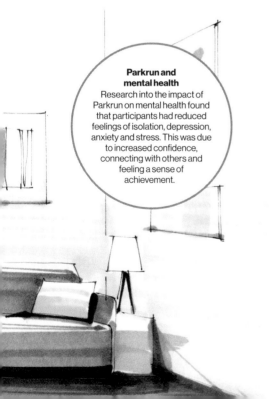

Parkrun and mental health
Research into the impact of Parkrun on mental health found that participants had reduced feelings of isolation, depression, anxiety and stress. This was due to increased confidence, connecting with others and feeling a sense of achievement.

REMOVE BARRIERS TO EXERCISE

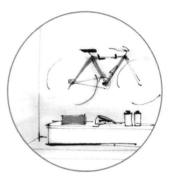

An accessible and organized place to keep your gear by the front door will make it easier to "grab and go" and put it away when you get home.

Wall-hanging bike storage fittings reduce hallway blockages and increase usable floorspace – just be careful after a muddy ride.

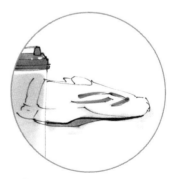

Remove the barriers to exercise by keeping your kit well maintained before you need to use it.

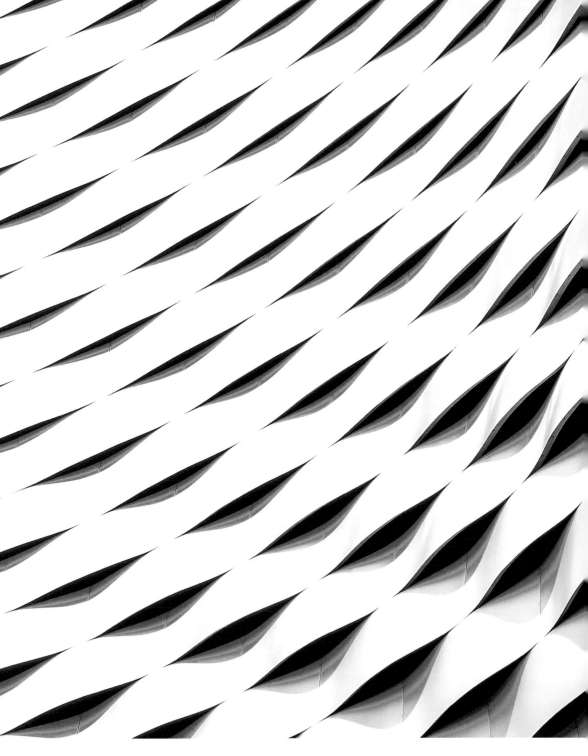

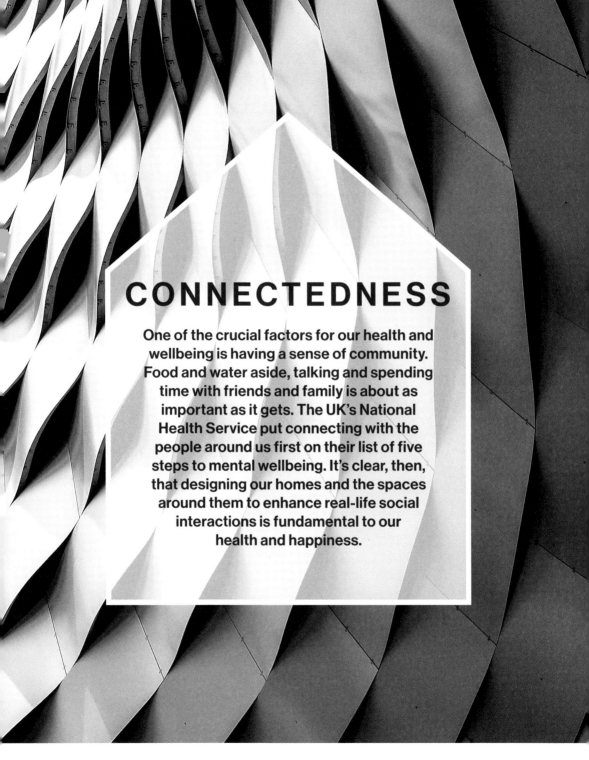

CONNECTEDNESS

One of the crucial factors for our health and wellbeing is having a sense of community. Food and water aside, talking and spending time with friends and family is about as important as it gets. The UK's National Health Service put connecting with the people around us first on their list of five steps to mental wellbeing. It's clear, then, that designing our homes and the spaces around them to enhance real-life social interactions is fundamental to our health and happiness.

25 | Make your kitchen inviting

The kitchen is the hub of the home for many. It is an active social space: we spend time here engaging with others, whether that's having a coffee or a glass of wine, cooking together or eating a meal with friends and family.

You can enhance these social opportunities by creating a diverse space with a dining table for eating, an island unit for perching at and alternative seating such as a sofa or armchair. Having low furniture will keep the space open and allow for sightlines through the space for maximum inclusivity; an open-plan layout is ideal for this and it can encourage people to gather and interact. However, if you prefer some separation between the kitchen and dining space, consider using semi-screening partitions, such as toughened glass, open shelving or planters to create soft boundaries rather than hard walls.

Of course, the importance of food and how it brings us together has a large role to play. A kitchen-diner should be somewhere that nourishes us and promotes healthy behaviours, and having the right kitchen equipment and food on display can go a long way towards this. Consider placing juicers or filtered water in an accessible space on the counter, or having an inviting fruit bowl or a kitchen herb box on the windowsill.

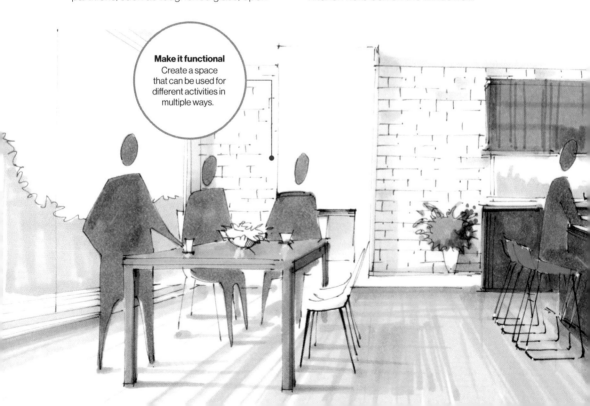

Make it functional
Create a space that can be used for different activities in multiple ways.

We can also use some of the benefits of colour (see pages 14–23): the kitchen could have vibrant pops of colour to energize us in the mornings and encourage upbeat socializing. Lighting is also key for enhancing social interactions. It is important to have a range of dimmable lighting to suit different functions and moods, from lively and open to romantic and intimate.

In other words, the kitchen and dining room should be adaptable, open and inviting spaces that create a perfect home hub where we want to spend time with others.

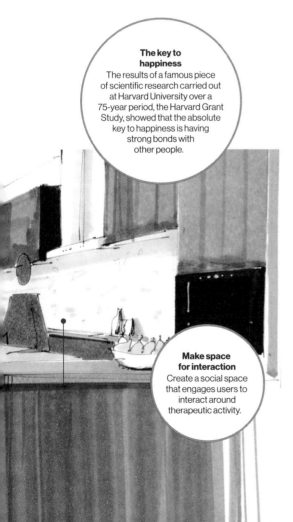

The key to happiness
The results of a famous piece of scientific research carried out at Harvard University over a 75-year period, the Harvard Grant Study, showed that the absolute key to happiness is having strong bonds with other people.

Make space for interaction
Create a social space that engages users to interact around therapeutic activity.

DISPLAY HEALTHY SNACKS

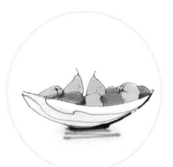

Place your kitchen herb box on a windowsill for accessible, fresh cooking ingredients.

Keeping a bowl of fruit on the counter not only looks nice, but it will remind you to reach for a healthy snack first.

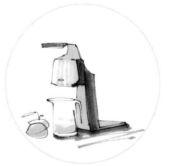

Keep a juicer on the counter to make juicing part of your routine rather than a chore.

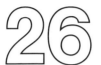

The power of soup

When it comes to lunchtime at the Oliver Heath Design studio, we gather to eat a bowl of fresh soup every day. At some point mid-morning, the question "what soup shall we make today?" will have arisen, resulting in a short deliberation and a quick trip to the nearby greengrocers.

The soup then gets made in our office kitchen by the volunteer of the day, and devoured around the meeting table amid much conversation and debate! We love this process so much that we make soup throughout the entire summer too, despite the heat. It feels wholesome and nourishing in more ways than one; we get health from our meal, and wellbeing from our sense of community.

How can you bring the power of soup into the home? Perhaps you could spend some time planning weekly meals with whomever you live with, giving each of you an opportunity to cook and share your favourite meal. Alternatively, get together and do some gardening, or try out each other's hobbies, whether that's a crafts evening or doing a puzzle. For some, conversation comes naturally as a way to connect, but for others it's easier to unite over the sharing of activities and skills.

The tip here is to dedicate space and furniture to allow these things to happen. Where can you store games so they're easily accessible? Is your table large and easy enough to clear to double up as an area to play or make? Have you created somewhere for others to sit with you while you cook, and is there enough counter space for them to join in? Are your craft or gardening tools organized and ready to go? If you want to stand the best chance of getting people to come together and join in, it really helps to work these things out in advance.

And perhaps most importantly, this space needs to be warm and inviting to draw people in and make them want to stay. Creating an atmosphere that enhances the quality of these moments could be as simple as lighting a fire, playing background music or bringing in extra cushions and throws.

Dedicate space and furniture that will help bring people together over shared activities and skills.

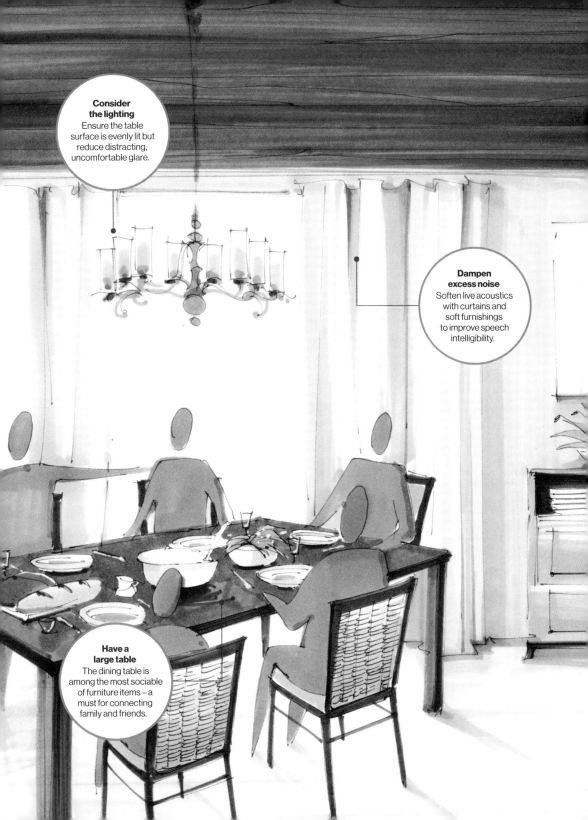

Consider the lighting
Ensure the table surface is evenly lit but reduce distracting, uncomfortable glare.

Dampen excess noise
Soften live acoustics with curtains and soft furnishings to improve speech intelligibility.

Have a large table
The dining table is among the most sociable of furniture items – a must for connecting family and friends.

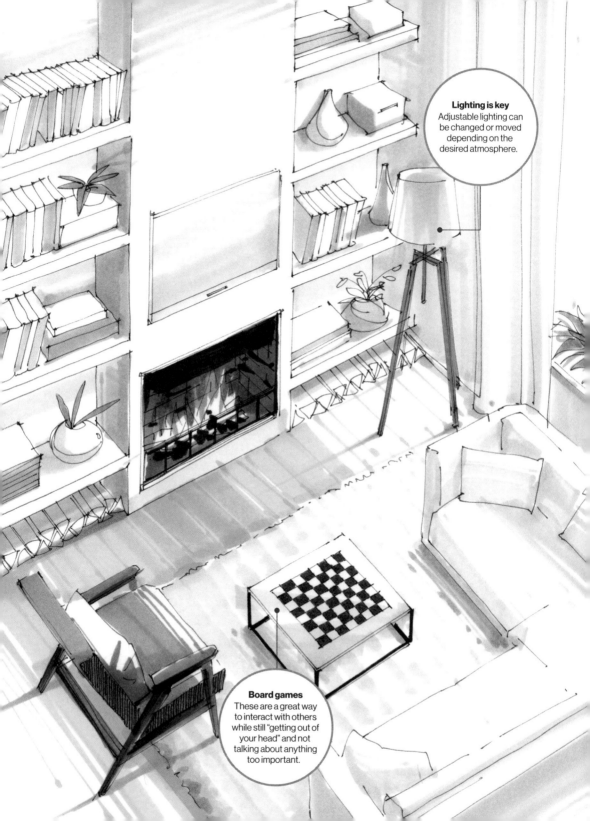

Lighting is key
Adjustable lighting can be changed or moved depending on the desired atmosphere.

Board games
These are a great way to interact with others while still "getting out of your head" and not talking about anything too important.

27 | Make your living space adaptable

The living room is another place where we spend time with others, but even when being sociable we still need moments of retreat to reset. Here, we spend time with others in a more passively social way. This space plays a very important role in supporting our mental wellbeing by allowing us to switch off and unwind while still enjoying quality time with our loved ones.

In the morning, we might spend some time in the living room with a morning coffee and a book or the newspaper. A high-backed armchair with a view outdoors is just the thing for this moment of peace.

We might also use the living room to be with others while watching TV, listening to music, gazing at the flickering flames of a fire or reading books in the evening. Your furniture arrangement can support this gentle social interaction – sofas and armchairs perpendicular to one another feel more relaxed than those that face each other directly, which can feel confrontational.

This space should be safe and contained, but also flexible, so it can adapt to our needs. Lively games or relaxed conversations with friends and family might happen here, so it's important that people have a sense of control. Lighting should be adjustable so that it can be changed to create different atmospheres. Similarly, having furniture that is moveable, such as a nest of small tables, will allow people to huddle around a coffee table or pull one over to rest a glass of wine.

Sofas and armchairs perpendicular to one another feel more relaxed than those that face each other directly.

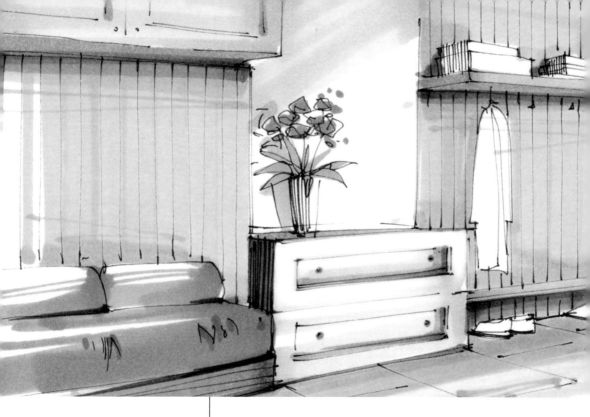

28 | Have a welcoming entrance way

Enjoying the external appearance of your house contributes to better mental wellbeing. The moment of transition as you enter the house should be a pleasant experience: a moment of decompression as you switch activities.

First impressions are important. Much of our first impression of a home is created as we approach the front door, so your welcome should start here. In fact, research has found that 80% of potential homebuyers decide whether or not a home is right for them as soon as they walk in.

Take a fresh look at the entrance way, flooring, greenery and the front door itself. Does it convey the welcome you would like? Repaving paths and updating flooring,

incorporating scented plants and greenery, adding a lick of fresh paint to front walls or the front door and installing a sensor-controlled light will make a dramatic difference, and welcome you or guests to your home.

Upon entering, this welcome will continue and develop, as your home's interior offers the first moments of personal expression. From a sensory side, it could include warm, welcoming colours, gentle scents from an atomizer, plants or flowers, and adjustable

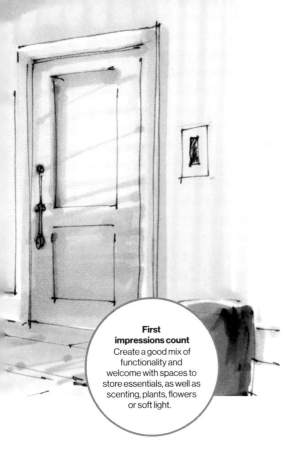

First impressions count
Create a good mix of functionality and welcome with spaces to store essentials, as well as scenting, plants, flowers or soft light.

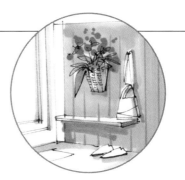

Have a seat to use by the front door for putting on and taking off shoes – no more wobbling around or blocking the stairs.

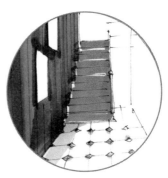

Use warm, welcoming colours in hardwearing finishes to create an inviting but practical space.

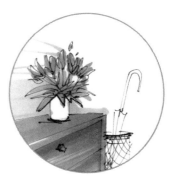

A display of plants or flowers by the front door will create a fresh, vibrant welcome as you enter the home.

lighting that can be soft and calming, or practical when it needs to be.

As this is a high-activity and functional space, be sure to paint walls in wipeable paints (eggshell or gloss) or durable patterned wallpapers to conceal marks and scuffs. Furniture should facilitate organization and preparedness to minimize stress as we enter or leave the home. Examples of this include a seat to put on and take off shoes, storage for shoes, hooks for coats and keys, and a mirror to check you're looking your best.

Conversations often happen in the hallway, as you enter and greet or say a chatty farewell while putting on shoes. While it may seem odd to suggest adding in seating here (you're hardly going to drink your cup of tea by the front door!), could that shoe storage double up as a seat to perch on?

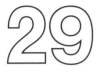

29 | Create focal points

Designing focal points in the home that draw people in to sit, admire, chat or relax, is a great way to bring people together and connect them. This creates shared emotional connections, which increases bonding and a sense of community.

Fire is an interesting example. From an evolutionary point of view, it has enabled us to stay warm, cook food and protect ourselves. This sense of safety has been carried into the present day; research suggests that we have lower blood pressure, form bonds with others and act more socially when we gather around a fire. This could be an open fireplace or wood-burning stove in the house (see page 140). If neither of those is an option, you could always play a video of a log fire on your TV or computer screen as an alternative.

You could also consider watching the sunset or stargazing. When we watch these with others, we feel connected. In the garden, you could create a well-lit, sheltered seating area with a firepit or chiminea, or a pergola with seating overlooking a view. Ideally, these outdoor spaces would be positioned where they aren't overlooked to create a relaxed setting for socializing.

Other focal points around the home could include a large-scale artwork, a water feature, a kinetic sculpture, a fish tank or any other eye-catching feature that could bring people together with joint attention, wonder and conversation.

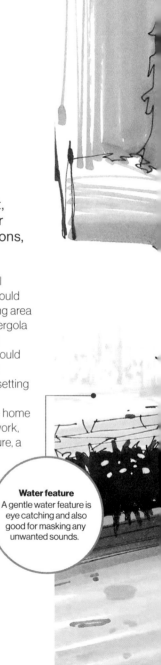

Water feature
A gentle water feature is eye catching and also good for masking any unwanted sounds.

Research suggests that we have lower blood pressure, form bonds with others and act more socially when we gather around a fire.

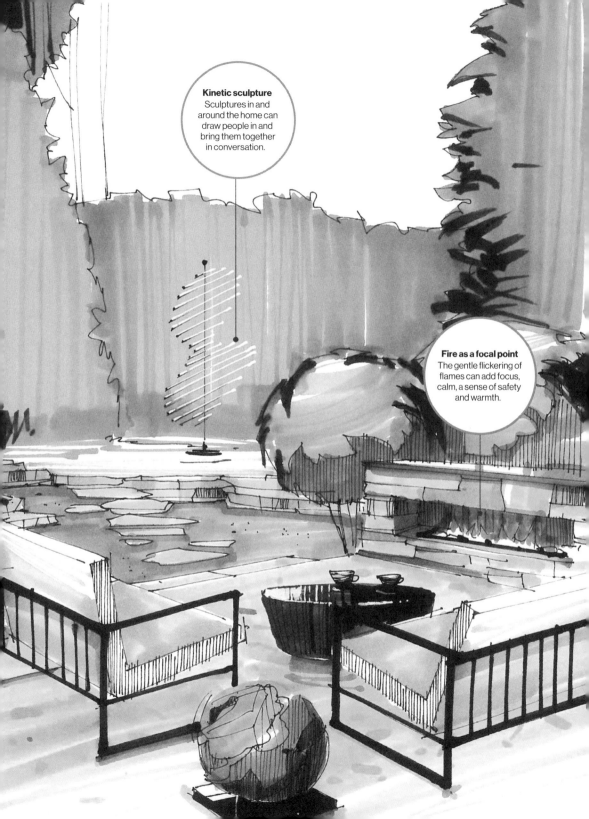

Kinetic sculpture
Sculptures in and around the home can draw people in and bring them together in conversation.

Fire as a focal point
The gentle flickering of flames can add focus, calm, a sense of safety and warmth.

30 Connect with your neighbours

Sociability and community don't only take place in the home. To feel fully content, having a good relationship with your neighbours is also important. Picture a scene where people are sitting out on their front porch and waving at passing neighbours, or inviting them in for a cup of coffee.

In the UK, sadly it's quite uncommon to know the people who live on our street. In fact, 8 out of 10 people here are concerned that our neighbourly relationships are waning. Perhaps it's the weather, or maybe we like to keep ourselves to ourselves more than some other cultures. But if we don't feel any sense of neighbourliness, we can end up feeling alienated, out of place and unsafe in our local areas.

Despite the decrease in neighbourliness over the years, a report by the Young Foundation found that 52% of people were happy to invite neighbours inside and 40% would trust their neighbour with a spare key. The potential is there; we might just need an opportunity.

The Young Foundation
This social innovator and non-profit think tank created a report on neighbourliness and belonging, which suggested that they can improve wellbeing, improve life chances, cut crime, help informal social control and facilitate mutual aid and support.

During the 2020 COVID-19 lockdown, many streets had their own mutual aid groups (created via social media platforms) so that neighbours could help each other with shopping and other errands. Groups like these, or the weekly nationwide doorstep round of applause to thank NHS workers, helped us connect with our neighbours.

It's possible to build on these experiences and foster connections with neighbours by creating spaces outside the front of your home where you can spend time. You might already have a garden to tend to, or some pot plants to water and prune regularly. Perhaps you could set up a bench out the front to catch the morning or evening sun. These are great ways to have incidental meetings with passing neighbours, which can be a lifeline for those who live alone.

TIPS FOR CONNECTING

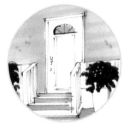

Add pot plants out front to tend to – you might just have a positive chance encounter with a neighbour.

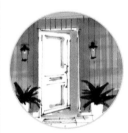

Good lighting by your front door enhances conversation and also improves security.

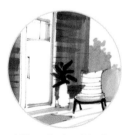

Add a seat or bench to sit on – this is a good way to have coffee with a neighbour.

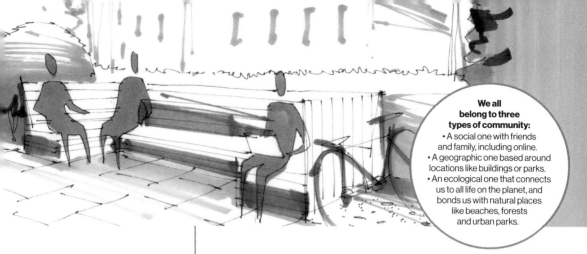

31 | Connect with the neighbourhood

Connecting with others in your area can enhance a sense of belonging and improve wellbeing. Neighbourhoods with greater social cohesion see lower rates of mental health problems, regardless of socioeconomic status.

But how do you go about this? In many warmer countries, the main square is an integral part of the community where, in the evenings, local people gather to talk and enjoy some fresh air in the cooler part of the day.

Although our climate isn't as well suited to these evening gatherings, there are other ways to connect with our local communities. A great starting point is to inhabit them, rather than going further afield: visiting the local park, restaurants and cafes, and shopping locally are great ways to get to know the area.

Many of us found a greater appreciation for our local nature spots during the 2020 lockdowns, and started exercising regularly in nearby outdoor spaces. These outdoor spaces must feel safe, and be attractive and easily accessible in order for this habit to continue to appeal. Community activities such as litter picking, seed bombing and community gardening can help, both by bringing people together in a shared activity and making the neighbourhood an attractive

place that people want to spend time in. In fact, research has found that mental wellbeing is better when we are happy with how our neighbourhood looks, and when we feel our home and local area are improving. If we believe our neighbourhood to be unattractive, we experience reduced wellbeing.

Parklets are a great addition to an urban neighbourhood. These are small pavement extensions for people to meet, stop and rest that often fill an empty parking space or two. They can be turned into mini parks with planting (hence the name). In some areas, they have increased foot traffic by 44%, tripled the number of people stopping by, and increased the perception of the area being fun, clean and sociable. So it doesn't take much! Perhaps there's a nearby space you know of that could be reclaimed in this way?

If you want to get involved, or even start one of these initiatives, there might be an online platform for meeting people in your area – and if there isn't one, you know what to do!

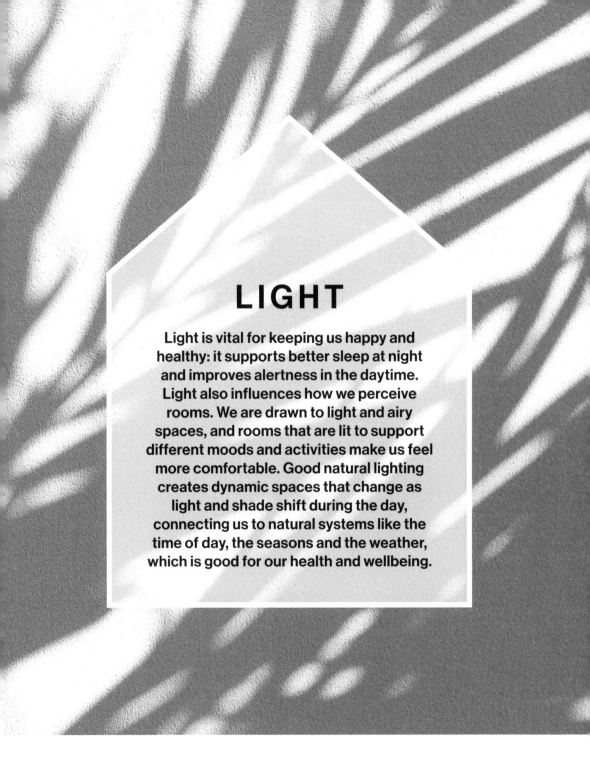

LIGHT

Light is vital for keeping us happy and healthy: it supports better sleep at night and improves alertness in the daytime. Light also influences how we perceive rooms. We are drawn to light and airy spaces, and rooms that are lit to support different moods and activities make us feel more comfortable. Good natural lighting creates dynamic spaces that change as light and shade shift during the day, connecting us to natural systems like the time of day, the seasons and the weather, which is good for our health and wellbeing.

32 | Get to know your circadian rhythms

We all have an internal body clock that roughly follows a 24-hour cycle according to the changes in light and darkness we experience throughout the day. This is known as our circadian rhythm, and it can be thrown out of kilter by things like travelling across time zones, staying up late or working night shifts, when artificial light extends the day's activities into the night.

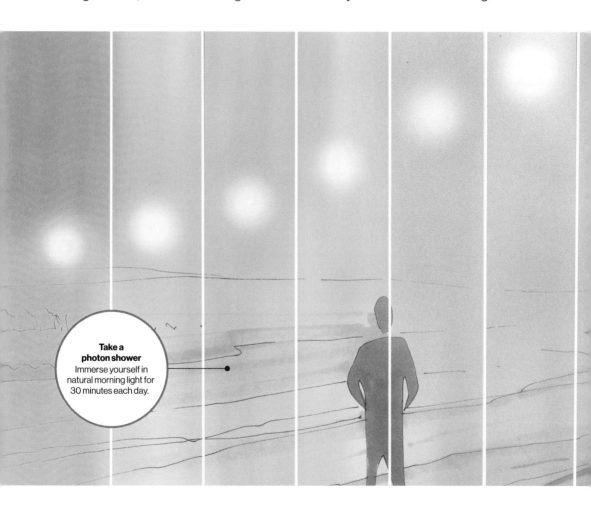

Take a photon shower
Immerse yourself in natural morning light for 30 minutes each day.

Circadian rhythms not only regulate our sleep cycles, but also affect behaviour, appetite, hormone release, body temperature and alertness. This explains why being tired can affect our mood, ability to focus and our food choices; we're more likely to eat unhealthily and gain weight when we are sleep deprived. Equally, poor sleep can make us grumpy, which can affect our relationships and adversely affect our concentration levels during the day.

Being aware of how our bodies respond to light is essential for creating a home that supports our health and happiness. Think about the times when you're functioning at your best, how and when tiredness affects you, how much time you spend outside and how much daylight you experience each day. Could your circadian rhythms be out of sync? In this section we'll show you how to use natural and artificial light to reset them and keep them healthy.

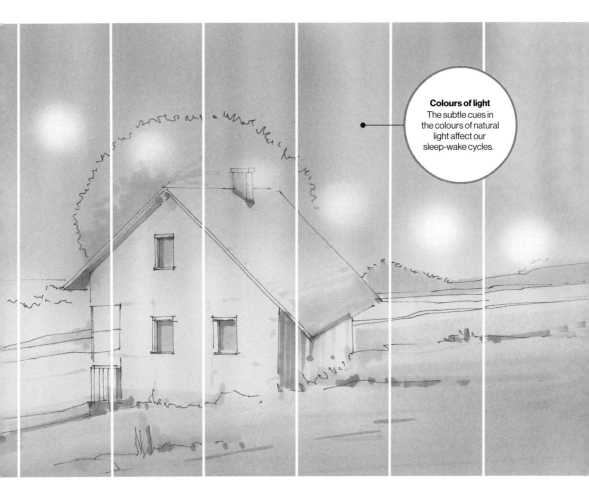

Colours of light
The subtle cues in the colours of natural light affect our sleep-wake cycles.

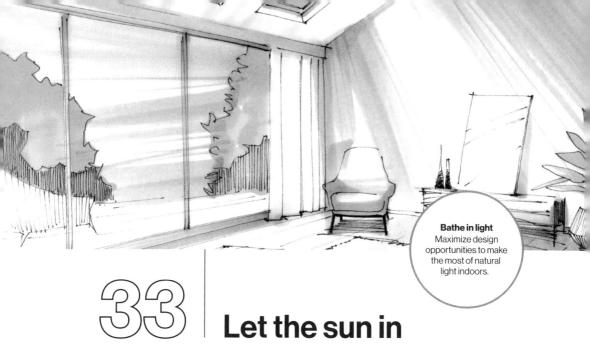

Bathe in light
Maximize design
opportunities to make
the most of natural
light indoors.

33 | Let the sun in

The easiest way to keep our circadian rhythms healthy is to increase our exposure to natural daylight. Since we spend around 90% of our lives indoors, it's important to allow in as much sunlight as possible. We might not have control over this at work, but we do at home.

Let's take a look at some of the things you can do outside to make sure nothing stops light coming in. Most simply, clean your windows. It's cheap and it makes an immediate difference to the quality of light in your home but is something we often forget.

Another great tip is to cut back foliage outside windows if it is blocking any light. Although having greenery in view is a good way to enhance wellbeing, we don't want it to be so close that it makes the room darker. This means keeping climbers tidy and bushes pruned. You might even consider lopping, trimming or cutting down an entire tree if you are living in its shadow. While we love trees and encourage them wherever possible, big trees too close to the house can be problematic (and beyond a certain height can nullify your home insurance policy). Ask a local tree surgeon to advise you on the best course of action.

MAXIMIZE NATURAL LIGHT

If you are undertaking a large design or refurbishment project, here are some things to consider:

Adding more windows, if planning permissions allow

Enlarging your windows by (most cost effectively) dropping the sills

Replacing existing windows with larger ones if you can, or choosing windows with smaller frames

Replacing the glass so that it is one solid piece rather than broken up by fenestration bars or leaded light strips

Adding a sun tube – a small reflective tube that lets light into windowless spaces near the roof, such as an upstairs corridor or stairwell

Adding a skylight to allow light to flood in, as well as aiding ventilation

34 | Make the most of sunlight

There are plenty of things you can do inside to make sure you're letting in as much sunlight as possible. Many people think that if they buy houseplants, a good place for them is the windowsill. Not true! A lot of plants don't like too much sunlight, and it blocks the light for you, who would benefit from it more.

Keeping your windows clear of obstruction from curtains and blinds is a good idea too. Curtains don't need to partially cover the window frame on either side. Consider fixing a slightly longer curtain rail, so your curtains can pull fully back, and perhaps you need tiebacks for your curtains to make sure they stay put. If you have blinds, the frame can sit above the window, so that's an option too.

The third tip might sound obvious, but if you have your sofa or bed with its back to the window, consider rotating it so it's facing the window instead. This way, you can make the most of the natural light by letting it all in, as well as being able to sit facing it. You might even have a nice view out, which has restorative benefits in itself.

Positioning houseplants away from windowsills will help let the light in.

KEEP YOUR WINDOWS CLEAR

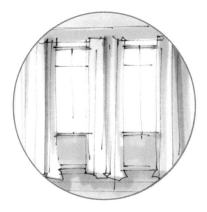

Fit your curtain rails to overshoot the window so you can pull your curtains back fully to let in all available natural light.

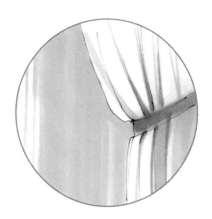

If you live in rented accommodation, you can add tiebacks to keep your curtains as open as possible.

35 | Get outside

Going outside does us the world of good. Research has found that sunlight exposure while camping, which is around 400% higher than normal daily levels, resets circadian rhythms.

Realistically, of course, most of us won't get that kind of exposure in our normal daily lives – but how about taking a photon shower? Circadian rhythm experts advise that one of the best ways to remedy a circadian rhythm that's out of sync is to experience an intense burst of natural light first thing in the morning, for around half an hour. If you take the opportunity to exercise outdoors, walk or cycle to work or even get outside just for pleasure, this will help rebalance your sleep/wake cycle.

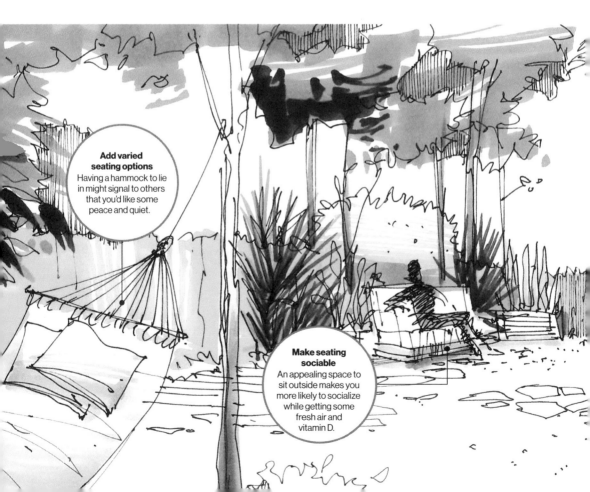

Add varied seating options
Having a hammock to lie in might signal to others that you'd like some peace and quiet.

Make seating sociable
An appealing space to sit outside makes you more likely to socialize while getting some fresh air and vitamin D.

When designing the home, it's also important to consider how we can encourage ourselves to go outside more. If you have a garden, you could create an easier flow from inside to outside by installing French doors or bi-folding doors, if you have the budget to do some remodelling. The idea is that we treat our outdoor space in the same way we treat indoor space: it should be inviting and draw us in. What opportunities are there for placemaking in the garden? Make the most of your outdoor space by creating lovely destination points you'll want to spend time sitting in. This might be a patio table and chairs, a hammock, a swinging chair, a sheltered area or a little reading nook.

Create lovely destination points that you want to spend time sitting in.

If you have a small balcony or terrace, put a chair out there with some pot plants to make it an easy and appealing place to go and sit instead of on your sofa.

Many of us don't have outdoor space, which means it's even more important to make the effort to find a nice nearby park to sit in on a sunny afternoon. At home, a comfortable seat next to an opening window can give you the burst of sunlight and fresh air you need.

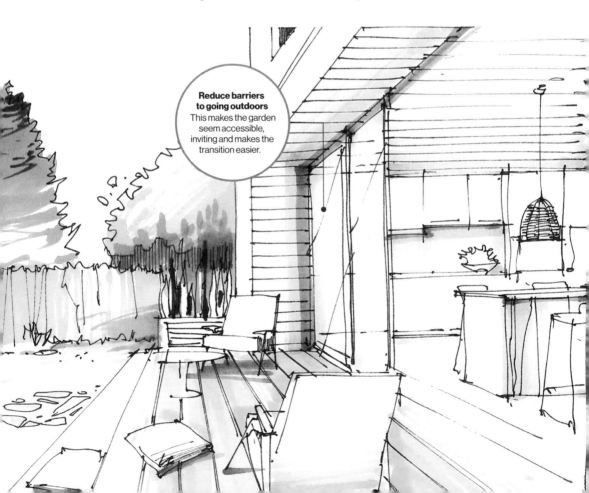

Reduce barriers to going outdoors
This makes the garden seem accessible, inviting and makes the transition easier.

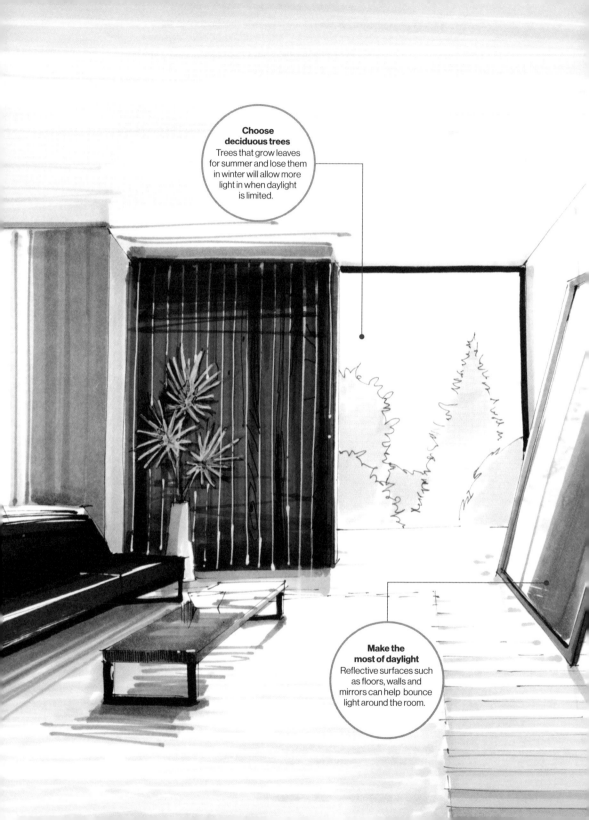

**Choose
deciduous trees**
Trees that grow leaves
for summer and lose them
in winter will allow more
light in when daylight
is limited.

**Make the
most of daylight**
Reflective surfaces such
as floors, walls and
mirrors can help bounce
light around the room.

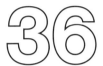

Maximize winter light

As winter approaches the days begin to get shorter and darker, which can throw our circadian rhythms off. We can be left feeling groggy while we get used to the new light cycle, and a little less than ecstatic that daylight hours are going to continue to decrease.

We adjust to the fatigue as our sleep-wake cycle catches up, but there are other longer-term mental health issues such as Seasonal Affective Disorder (SAD) to deal with throughout the dark winter months, when we are spending more time than ever indoors. It is thought that a lack of sunlight stops the hypothalamus (a small part of the brain that regulates important functions, including circadian rhythms) from working properly, which leads to a lack of serotonin (the "happy hormone") and a disrupted body clock. Seasonal Affective Disorder is estimated to affect 10 million Americans, and another 10–20% of the population are thought to have it mildly. This quite clearly illustrates how important light is for our health and wellbeing, and how sensitive we are to changes in the amount we get. Hopefully you can now see the importance of making the most of the limited amount of daylight during the winter months.

Inside, light is reflected and absorbed differently by different surfaces and textures. If walls and furnishings in your home are dark in colour, they will absorb the light. Consider maximizing any light you can get into your space by using lighter-coloured surfaces, reflective paints, glazed tiles and mirrors. These bounce the light around the room and make the space feel brighter and bigger.

Having deciduous trees outside, which lose their leaves in winter and grow them in summer, is a great way to let light come through when it is needed most – and they offer shade when it is not.

Research has shown that the switch to DST (Daylight Saving Time) has been linked to increased injuries, car accidents and depression.

Prevent glare

Natural light is dynamic; there are varying densities of light and shadow that move and change throughout the day, which means they will move around your home too. At certain times of day, you have some areas that are very sunny. Although letting that sunlight in can have an amazing effect on your health and wellbeing, too much can become a hindrance.

Glare from sunlight can either be direct or reflected off bright surfaces, and can cause major discomfort, headaches and even eye damage. Spend some time observing how the light comes into your house throughout the seasons to identify where glare may be a problem. If it is an issue, here are some ideas to diffuse or prevent glare from natural light.

> **Glare from sunlight or reflective surfaces can cause major discomfort, headaches and even eye damage.**

TIPS FOR PREVENTING GLARE

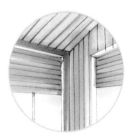

Fit adjustable window-blinds to offer more control.

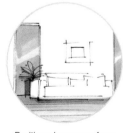

Position mirrors away from windows that get direct sun.

Place films on windows to reflect or reduce sunlight.

Use darker, more absorbent paints, furniture and furnishings in bright spots.

Replace a transparent conservatory roof with a solid insulated roof with skylights.

Change the position of furniture that has reflective surfaces, such as glass tabletops.

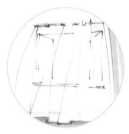

Use sheer materials or curtains on windows.

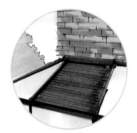

Fit controllable blinds on a conservatory roof or skylight.

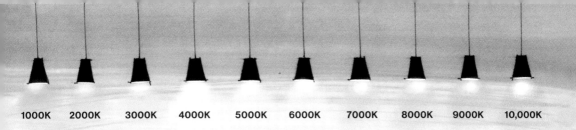

1000K 2000K 3000K 4000K 5000K 6000K 7000K 8000K 9000K 10,000K

Cool or warm?
Cool white bulbs (4000K or more) are bright and stimulating; warm white (around 3000K) is welcoming; a candle is around 1900K.

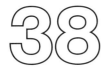

Get artificial lighting right

Once you've done what you can to improve natural light, it's time to consider artificial lighting. Getting the right amount and quality of electric light will help you to navigate around your home and undertake the tasks you need to do; to function better, by maintaining your sleep/wake cycle; and to feel better, by connecting you more deeply to spaces and the people in them.

Over the years, we have become used to understanding lighting measured in watts, from the old incandescent warm yellow tungsten bulbs. As technology has advanced, we have more energy-efficient, brighter and longer-lasting bulbs, which measure lighting levels in lux or lumens.

There is also colour temperature to consider, measured in Kelvin or K. This measures the colour of light across the colour spectrum, which will have an impact on your body's physiological response to it.

In our multifunctional homes, we will need different types of light at different times of day for different moods or tasks. All spaces in the house should have different lighting options so that they can be adapted to fit your needs. This should include:
• **Good general (or ambient) lighting** to aid circulation around the house. This could be dimmable spotlighting so it can be bright for activities and dimmed later in the day.

• **Task lighting**, such as side lamps, standing lamps and spotlights above or next to specific task areas.
• **Mood or accent lighting** for hosting or simply relaxing.

Consider how you want to feel and how much light you will need for each activity in each space, and then choose the right type of lighting for each. Dimmable or even colour-changing options will add flexibility, which increases a beneficial sense of control and our needs being met.

All spaces in the house should have different lighting options so that they can be adapted to fit your needs.

Furniture position
Orientate the furniture layout to maximize views out of a window and enjoy dusk or early morning light.

39 | Introduce circadian lighting

Based on what we know about circadian rhythms (see page 70), it follows that keeping the lighting indoors close to the natural light outside is important for both our physical and mental health. We can do this in the home by making sure the colour of the lighting reflects the time of day as much as possible.

Circadian lighting, in essence, follows a "sunrise to sunset" cycle, according to which lights should be brighter and bluer in the morning (blue light makes us feel alert), and warmer orange light that mimics dusk to facilitate sleep should be used in the evening. Circadian lighting might seem complicated if you've never heard of it before, but it can be done in a number of easy ways.

At its simplest, try using a string of very warm white, or orange, LEDs (light emitting diodes) in the evening when you are relaxing before bedtime.

In overhead or side lights, use circadian light bulbs, which can be set to different colours of light using your existing light switch (the colour is controlled by the number of times you press the switch).

Use colour-changing LED light strips or bulbs with their own colour remote controller (these can easily be found in DIY shops or at online retailers).

Consider buying colour-changing lighting products, such as stand-alone table or floor lamps.

Use a wake-up light alarm clock to wake you gently with colour-changing lights in the morning, and relax you with soft lighting in warm tones at bedtime.

Keeping the lighting indoors close to the natural light outside is important for both our physical and mental health.

General lighting
This should be on a dimmer to reduce glare and soften the space.

Soft bedside lighting
Colour-adjustable bedside lights can enhance sleep when set to a dusk-like orange.

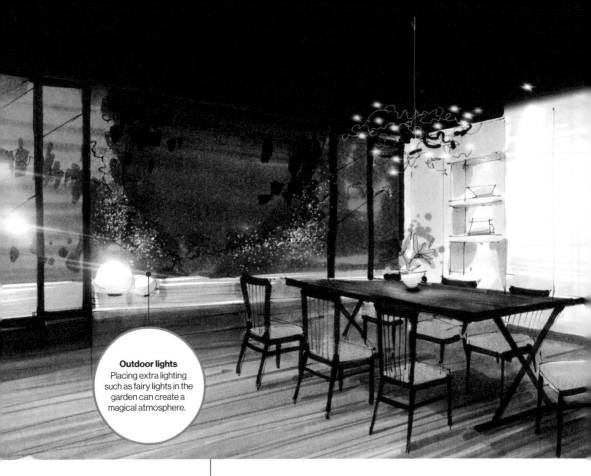

Outdoor lights
Placing extra lighting such as fairy lights in the garden can create a magical atmosphere.

40 | Add some magic touches

Last but definitely not least, adding some final special touches can really make a space feel complete and inviting, and add a sense of wonder.

You might want to put up some fairy lights behind your sofa, bed or along a mantelpiece, or put them in an orange-tinted glass jar to turn on at night for a warm, cosy glow. Fairy lights in garden trees or bushes never go amiss when entertaining.

Other ideas include firelight (in the home, or as a fire pit in the garden), a rotating lamp that projects light, or a lampshade with cut-outs that cast shadows or patterns onto the walls and ceiling. You could even use a projector to create beams of light through the space and onto surrounding walls in whatever colours and patterns you desire. Consider hanging a disco ball where it will catch the light at certain times of day, or a rainbow maker or rainbow-making glass film on the window too.

The movement of these forms of lighting

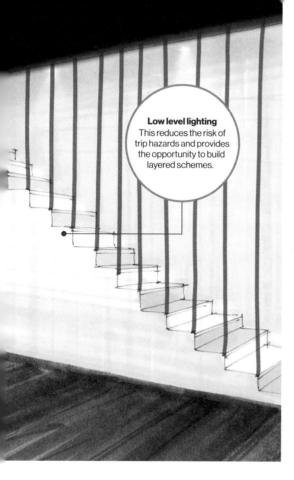

Low level lighting
This reduces the risk of trip hazards and provides the opportunity to build layered schemes.

can add an extra natural dimension called non-rhythmic sensory stimuli or NRSS (see page 43) to the space, which is more dynamic and restorative than regular, fixed lighting.

If you have the budget, you could even install small LED ceiling lights that are reminiscent of a twinkling, starry night sky, as you might sometimes find in a spa. In windowless rooms, you might consider investing in LED virtual skylights and light panels to create an illusion of there being a window with a blue sky behind. There are some very sophisticated systems that can create this, so have a look. These are just some of the magic touches you can consider to increase the sense of wonder and wellbeing in your home.

SPECIAL TOUCHES WITH LIGHTING

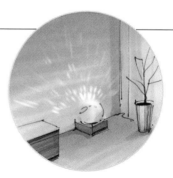

A disco ball or rainbow maker can reflect light magically around the room – it will change with movement and the position of the sun.

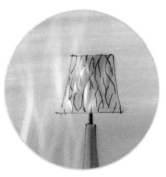

A lampshade with cut-outs can cast shadows onto the walls and ceiling if paired with a clear glass bulb.

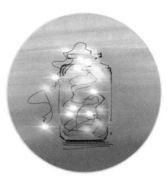

Fairy lights in a jar can add charm and a warm, cosy glow.

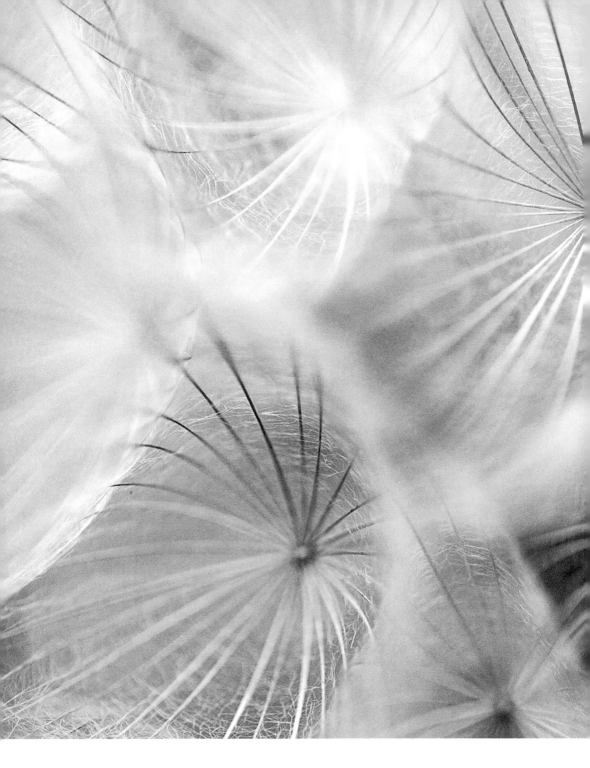

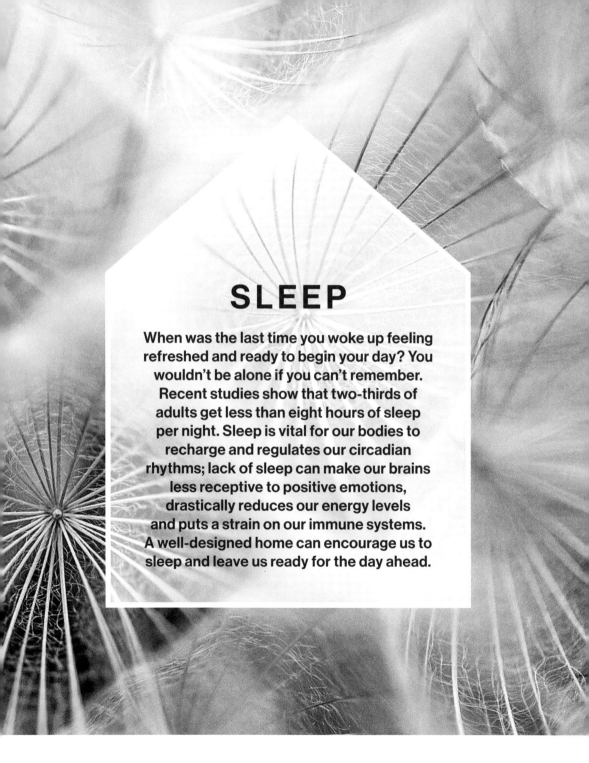

SLEEP

When was the last time you woke up feeling refreshed and ready to begin your day? You wouldn't be alone if you can't remember. Recent studies show that two-thirds of adults get less than eight hours of sleep per night. Sleep is vital for our bodies to recharge and regulates our circadian rhythms; lack of sleep can make our brains less receptive to positive emotions, drastically reduces our energy levels and puts a strain on our immune systems. A well-designed home can encourage us to sleep and leave us ready for the day ahead.

Design a bedroom retreat

Our bedrooms should provide us with a space for retreat, rest and recuperation. How can we make sure we wake up feeling refreshed and ready for the day? Here are some design features that can help remind our brains that it's time to drift off.

We perceive 80% of our built environment through our eyes, so it's important to recognize the visual impact the bedroom has. Colours should be calming and tonal in range, allowing the eyes to shift effortlessly from one colour to the next without it being jarring. Darker colours can work well in the bedroom, if you want to create a cave- or womb-like feeling (see page 23 for tips on this). Patterns should be nature-inspired and gentle, as these are proven to help us relax.

Furniture layout should prioritize the bed, creating a focal point and a sense of calming function to the room. Add variety with a chaise longue, window seat or armchair to encourage conversation or relaxation in other ways. Soft, inviting fabrics layered up on beds or furniture, whether in the form of pillows, cushions or throws, create a welcoming space that beckons you to relax.

Our sense of touch is closely linked to our emotions. Natural materials can feel authentic and nurturing, and promote a sense of warmth; a weighted wool blanket can make a child feel protected and secure; the tufted quality of a carpet on our feet can feel relaxing and soft. If you have bare floorboards, consider introducing a textural rug to soften and warm your journey to and from bed.

When choosing furniture and furnishings for your bedroom, focus on their tactile qualities and how they make you feel. Try closing your eyes and running your hands over them to decide if they're right for your space.

Finally, surround yourself with things that remind you of happy times spent in nature – perhaps a shell collection, a bowl of pinecones or a picture frame made from driftwood you found by the shore.

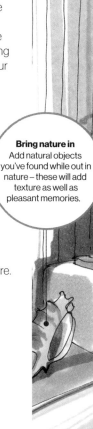

Bring nature in
Add natural objects you've found while out in nature – these will add texture as well as pleasant memories.

Colours should be calming and tonal in range, allowing the eyes to shift effortlessly from one colour to the next.

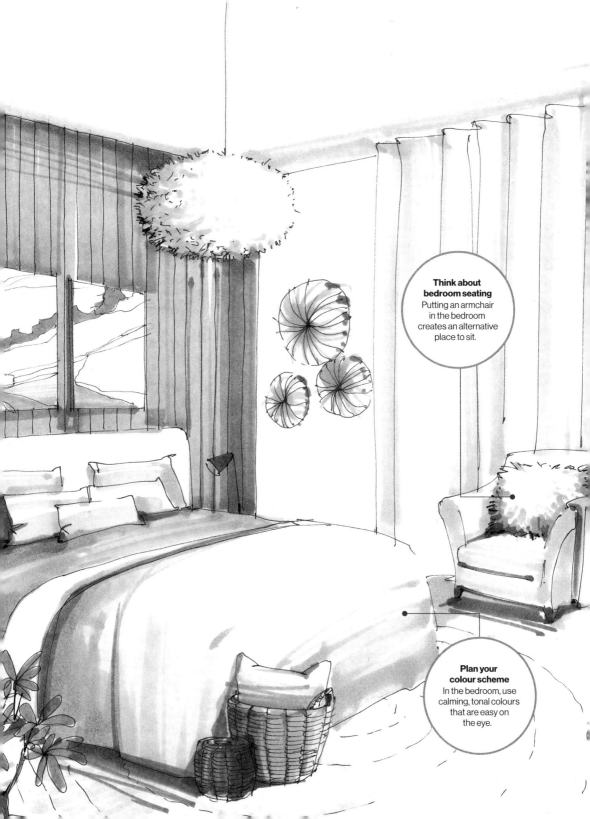

**Think about
bedroom seating**
Putting an armchair
in the bedroom
creates an alternative
place to sit.

**Plan your
colour scheme**
In the bedroom, use
calming, tonal colours
that are easy on
the eye.

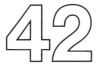

Create darkness

During the summer months, sunlight can leak into our bedrooms far earlier than we would like it to. This can disrupt our circadian body clocks and leave us feeling groggy and unrested.

Our bodies are programmed to associate darkness with rest and light with being awake. Sudden bright lights send messages to the brain, causing it to release hormones that make it harder to fall back to sleep. Ensuring your bedroom is dark at night will help improve the quality of your sleep and get you drifting off with ease. Here are some ways of preventing excess light from entering the room.

First, do a quick survey of your bedroom and try to spot any unwanted light sources that are filtering through. Common culprits could be street lamps, security lighting, porch lights, electronic alarm clocks and chargers. The window is an obvious source of light, so consider fitting some high-quality blackout curtains. These can reduce external noise as well as cutting down the glare of unwanted light. Wooden shutters and venetian blinds are also designed to help block out unwanted light. These traditional systems are adaptable to suit your needs, and can be retracted fully to allow light in when you want it.

If other members of your household stay up later than you and light is leaking through under your door, you could place a draft excluder over the gap.

Our bodies are programmed to associate darkness with rest and light with being awake.

ENSURING YOUR BEDROOM IS DARK

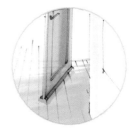

Place a draft excluder in the gap under your door if other household members have the lights on in the rest of the house after you go to bed.

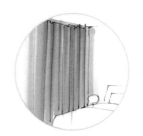

Blackout curtains will ensure no unwanted light enters the bedroom.

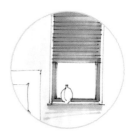

Wooden shutters can also reduce some light while letting in some of it in the morning if you prefer to be woken naturally.

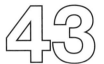

Reduce visual clutter

Did you know that tidying your room can lead to a better night's sleep? One study found that women who described their houses as cluttered had higher levels of the stress hormone cortisol, and found it harder to "switch off" at night. Living in untidiness keeps the mind active, as it visually reminds us that we have things to do. Here are some tips to help keep your room clutter free.

First, remove any items associated with your work life from your bedroom, such as laptops, paperwork or notes. These are visual cues to think about work and keep the mind ticking. Choose relaxing artwork, and remove any intense, chaotic scenes. Given the chance, our brains like to work things out and analyse, but calm and conceptual imagery that allows for soft attention can help our minds to wander.

Under-bed storage is also a great way to visually reduce clutter, as is a wardrobe with drawers rather than a clothes rail or open shelving. If you like to have selected treasured items on display, consider colour-coordinating those pieces and use uniform hangers to create rhythm. Finally, donate unwanted items to charity shops every once in a while to free up space and give clothes a new lease of life.

> **Living in untidiness keeps the mind active, as it visually reminds us that we have things to do.**

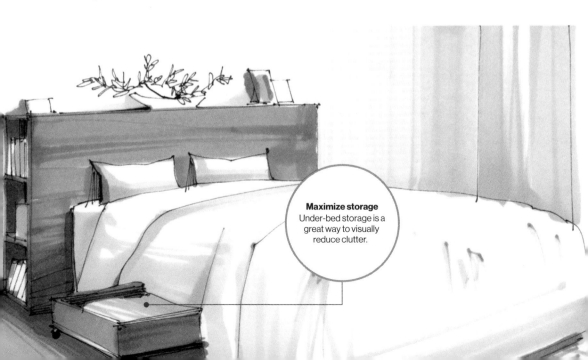

Maximize storage
Under-bed storage is a great way to visually reduce clutter.

44 | Choose a good mattress

A good-quality mattress will support you while you rest, and help you avoid serious health conditions like chronic back pain. Mattresses come in many sizes, materials and construction methods. Here are the pros and cons of the most popular types.

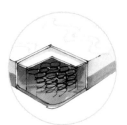

Open spring

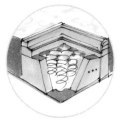

Pocket spring

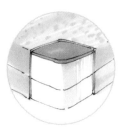

Memory foam

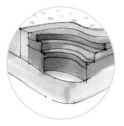

Latex

Open-spring mattresses consist of metal coils forged into springs, with a perimeter coil holding its shape together. They are great value, but are much less supportive than other mattress types and need replacing more often. Consider using them in guest bedrooms where they will get less use.

The pocket-spring mattress is a more supportive choice, as each spring is individually housed in its own pocket of fabric. They are well suited to couples sharing a bed, as the individual springs help balance the spread of different weights.

Both open-spring and pocket-spring mattresses are more breathable than latex or memory foam mattresses. However, they are often filled with materials such as lamb's wool that can trap dust. Whether or not you have allergies, remember to vacuum them regularly.

Memory foam is a mouldable material that reacts to temperature and weight. This makes it comfortable and ideal if you have a bad back, as it relieves pressure on sore joints and muscles. They can be quite heavy and hot, which some people find uncomfortable in summer. However, they are made of hypoallergenic materials, so are great for allergy sufferers.

Latex mattresses are ideal for people who like a supportive mattress but get hot during the night. Latex is a natural material made from the sap of rubber trees; it is very springy, breathable and resistant to mould and dust mites. It maintains its shape well, encouraging natural spine alignment.

When your mattress arrives, let it air in a well-ventilated space for a few hours to allow any toxins to be released.

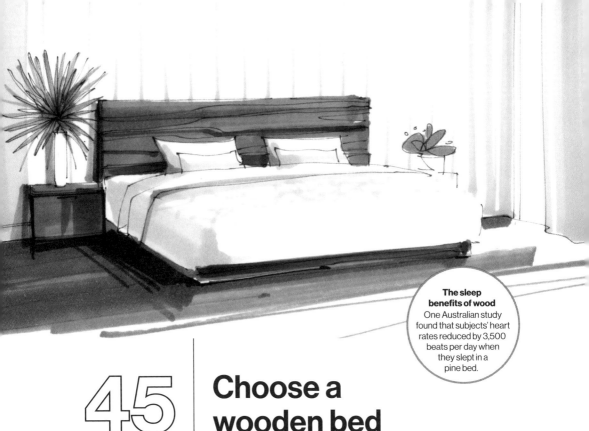

45 | Choose a wooden bed

We have seen that humans have an inherent attraction to timber (see page 32), and we find its presence comforting and calming. It seems that investing in a timber bed frame may well contribute to getting a good night's sleep.

Aside from the health benefits, it's hard to argue against the beauty of a timber bed, and it has functional advantages too. For starters, timber furniture helps moderate indoor air quality; the timber absorbs moisture in humid environments and releases moisture in dry conditions, thus keeping the moisture levels balanced.

In terms of air quality, wooden beds are easier to wipe and clean than beds with fabric headboards, which can collect dust, which in turn leads to dust mites. Wooden beds are also sturdy and don't squeak as much, which can be appealing if you're a light sleeper. This sturdiness keeps the bed functional and ergonomic, with a good headboard that you can comfortably rest up against while drinking a morning coffee or reading before sleep. We've all experienced the annoyance of pillows slipping through cold, metal poles!

A well-crafted timber bed can last you a lifetime. In this sense, it is an environmentally friendly choice. Just remember to check that the wood is from a sustainable source and is certified by the Forest Stewardship Council (FSC).

It's also worth checking that your bed frame doesn't contain any harmful "off-gassing" substances that can release toxins (see page 155 for more information on this).

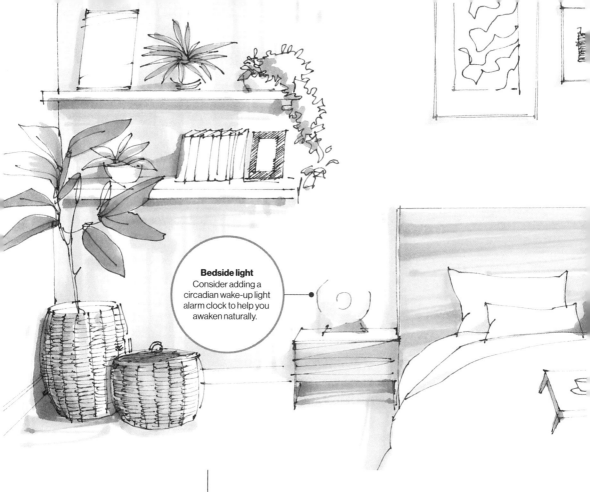

Bedside light
Consider adding a circadian wake-up light alarm clock to help you awaken naturally.

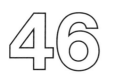

46 | Think about bedroom lighting

Having seen the importance of circadian rhythms (see page 70), we need to be particularly mindful when choosing bedroom lighting. Getting this right will help you get to sleep more readily and wake feeling more refreshed.

First, to help your body navigate into a peaceful slumber, you should remove electronic devices from your bedroom. As our modern world has become increasingly digitalized, so has our exposure to screens before bedtime. The blue light that is emitted from screens has shorter wavelengths and suppresses the production of melatonin, the hormone that induces sleep, whereas red light doesn't have this effect.

If you must have a phone in your room, set it to night time mode in the evening, if it has one.

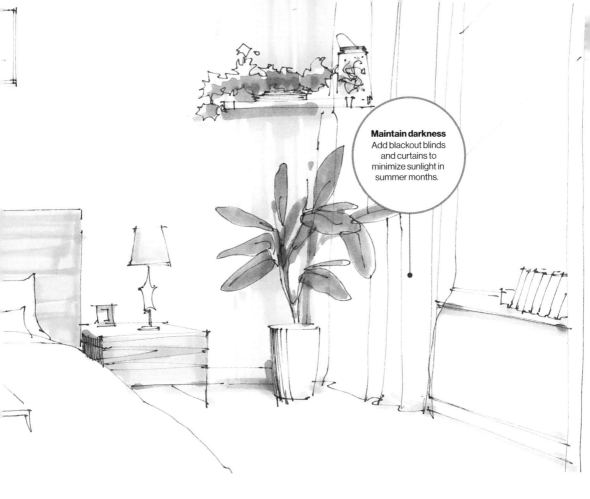

Maintain darkness
Add blackout blinds
and curtains to
minimize sunlight in
summer months.

Reading is a common bedtime ritual, but e-book readers should also be adjusted to a warm light setting.

Secondly, invest in reading or bedside lights that have a dimmer and colour control, which allows them to be set to a deep, warm, dusk-like colour before you sleep. Try not to rely on one singular pendant light in the centre of your ceiling, as this won't allow for flexible lighting options.

Bedside clocks are available that have integral colour-changing circadian lighting that echoes the daylight outside. This allows you to drift off to sleep and wake up to more natural-feeling light. We can't recommend them highly enough.

Invest in reading or bedside lights that have a dimmer and colour control.

Finally, consider your journey to bed and the lighting levels you experience along the way. If you have an en-suite bathroom, for example, think about fitting ambient furniture lighting. This could take the form of built-in LED light strips under your vanity cabinet or behind your mirror, producing a warm glow that doesn't shock you awake when you're winding down (or in the middle of the night!).

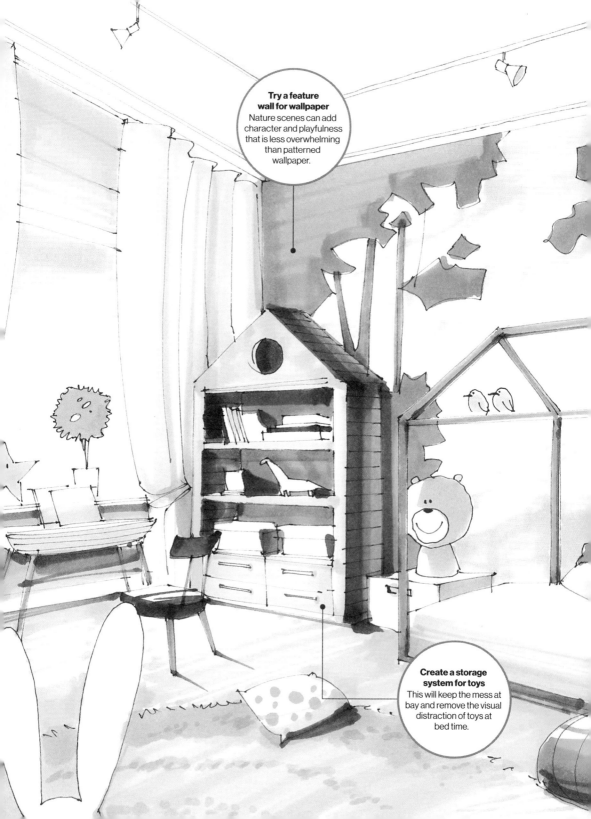

Try a feature wall for wallpaper
Nature scenes can add character and playfulness that is less overwhelming than patterned wallpaper.

Create a storage system for toys
This will keep the mess at bay and remove the visual distraction of toys at bed time.

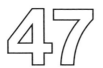 # Create healthy children's rooms

Designing a child's bedroom that can evolve with them as they grow takes some careful planning. Other than providing a space for sleep, it should also function as somewhere they can play, socialize and learn. With some simple design solutions you can create a room that adapts to your child's needs over the years.

Children need a space to be creative, process the world and have an escape. Aside from opting for hardwearing, wipeable surfaces that withstand arts and crafts, think about building a magical den or retreat in the corner of the room. This could be with ambient lighting, such as fairy lights and a fabric pop-up indoor tent.

When it's time to put the toys away, a good storage system is at the top of the list for maintaining a tidy, flexible space. If you're limited on space, choose storage that can double up as seating, such as chests or upholstered window seats. Consider using closed storage systems for items that aren't used as often and save the open storage for favourite toys or precious objects. Adjustable shelves are also a great choice for when old toys find new homes, as you can adapt them to hold books and photo frames.

Shutters, heavy curtains and blackout blinds can prevent sleep disturbances, and are also a great opportunity to interject fun textures and colour. Further textural inputs such as soft, weighted blankets can offer a sense of protection and keep your child snoozing for longer.

Wallpaper and paint colour can add personality and character to a room. Sometimes, although children's wallpaper is fun and playful, it can be quite busy and feel overwhelming. If you do opt for wallpaper, consider using it on just one feature wall, or choose one with neutral tones and stimulating textures instead. Selecting a calming and neutral colour scheme will help children relax and it won't date so easily. When selecting your paints, choose zero or ultra-low VOC ranges, as these are the healthiest option for air quality.

Although children's wallpaper is fun and playful, it can be quite busy and feel overwhelming.

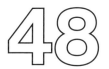 Regulate your temperature

It's important to make sure you're the right temperature at night to get a good sleep. Surprisingly, the best temperature for this is different from when we are awake. During the day, the average room temperature is around 20°C, but at night the ideal temperature is around 18°C .

Our bodies can overheat more quickly in the night, so falling asleep with the heating on, however tempting, can result in some tossing and turning. Scientists have found that people with insomnia tend to have a higher temperature at bedtime, which can make sleep a struggle.

First, regulate your bedroom temperature more accurately by installing a thermostatic radiator valve (see page 139). These are great in the bedroom because they sense the air temperature in the room and, when the desired temperature is reached, adjust the hot water flow, so you won't risk overheating.

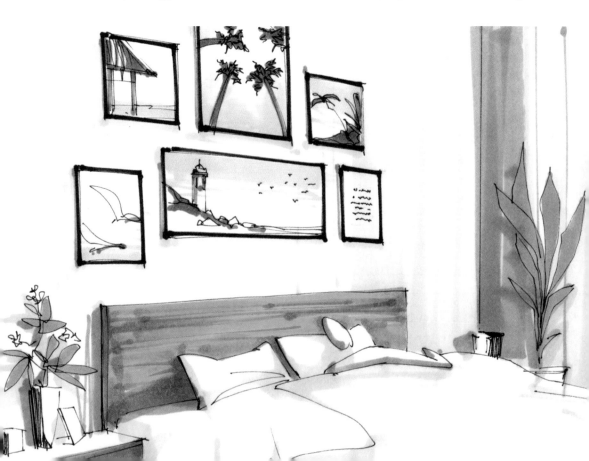

Second, consider temperature-regulating bedding such as wool duvets, or split-tog "partner" duvets if you have different temperature needs from the person you sleep with. Wool is breathable and self-regulating, keeping you cool or warm as required. It is also self-wicking, so it can draw moisture away from you if you sweat at night due to heat. This traditional technology has so far mostly been used in outerwear, but is now making its way into the bedroom.

Finally, in the heat of summer we often reach for a fan to help us keep cool at night. Fans are perfectly acceptable, but look for one with a Quiet Mark award label (see page 109 for more on this), which means their mechanical whirring noise shouldn't disturb your sleep.

(see page 109 for more on this)

HEAT REGULATION TIPS

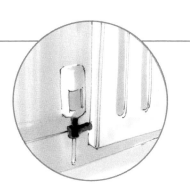

Thermostatic radiator valves can sense the air temperature and adjust the flow of hot water to the radiator accordingly.

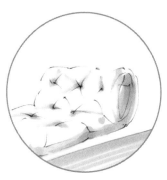

Wool is a breathable material for duvets and blankets, and can draw moisture away from your body at night.

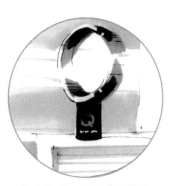

Look for a fan with the Quiet Mark label on it so that you won't be kept awake on hot summer nights.

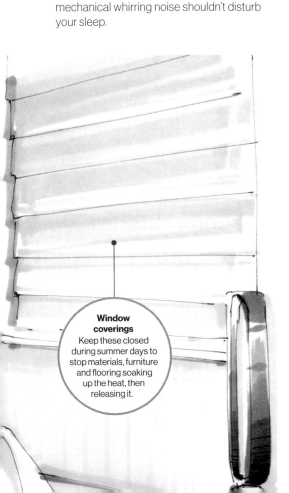

Window coverings
Keep these closed during summer days to stop materials, furniture and flooring soaking up the heat, then releasing it.

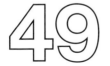

Create
bedtime rituals

After a long day, switching off at night can be hard and, as we already know, many people struggle with sleep disorders. It's good to have a regular routine that helps you unwind on your journey towards sleep.

First, avoid screens for at least an hour before bed. Instead, you might have a book or a journal on your bedside table. Writing down the events of the day, a to-do list for tomorrow and any other worry or idea that comes to mind as you get into bed can help to de-clutter your mind and allow you to leave it until the morning. Accompany this soothing activity with herbal tea in your favourite mug, such as valerian root, lavender or chamomile.

For extra relaxation, using a weighted blanket has been proven to enhance feelings of security and calm. While it might not be for everyone, the pressure from the blanket stimulates the relaxation hormone serotonin, which allows us to get to sleep faster

and have better-quality rest.

Consider practising some type of calming breathing exercise, which can be aided with a mindfulness or mediation app to guide you through the process. This does mean looking at your phone or tablet screen briefly, but the benefits may outweigh the negatives in this case.

Listening to nature sounds and using natural scent can also be part of your bedtime routine (see pages 113 and 158). And if you can, try to go to bed at the same time each night. That way, your body clock will know it's time to switch off and get some rest.

Try a weighted blanket
These have been shown to increase serotonin and the sleep hormone melatonin, as well as reducing cortisol.

Writing down the events of the day or a to-do list for tomorrow as you go to bed can help declutter your mind.

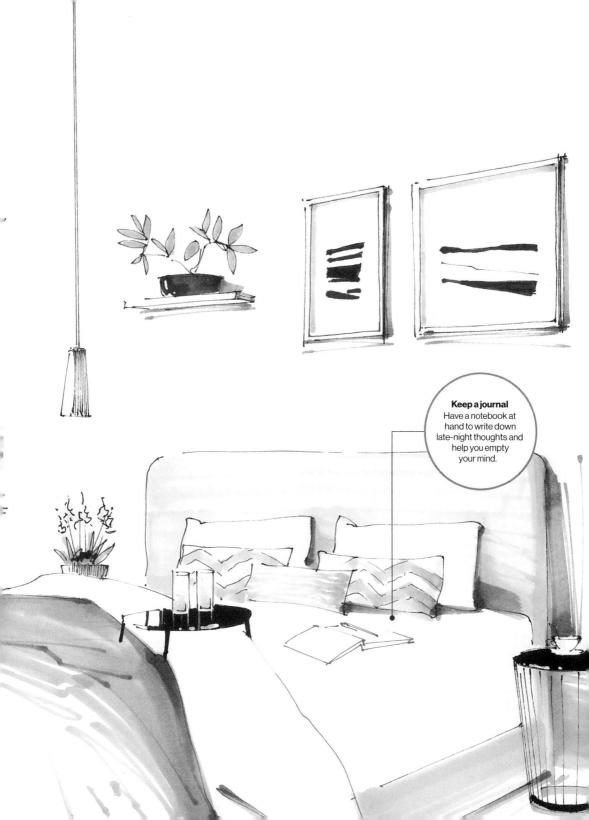

Keep a journal
Have a notebook at hand to write down late-night thoughts and help you empty your mind.

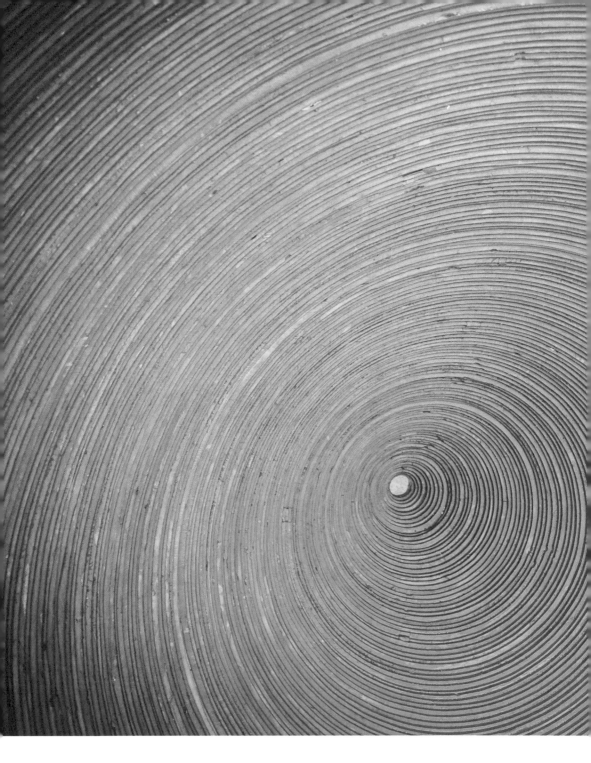

SOUND

Our hearing is much more important to our wellbeing than we may realize. In the distant past, it helped us hear approaching predators and locate prey. It's also vital for spatial awareness and communicating with others. These days, the acoustic landscape is often dominated by mechanical sounds that bounce off buildings and streets, and noise pollution can affect our sleep, increase hypertension and impact on our ability to concentrate and function well. So it's clear that we need to consider how to improve the acoustics in our homes.

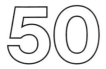

50 | Choose sound or silence

Which is best for wellbeing, sound or silence? It depends on who you ask; each of us has a different auditory threshold. This means that people need different levels of sound in their environment, and the wrong level can make us feel either under- or over-stimulated, affecting our stress levels.

The fact that there will be people with different thresholds in one household complicates things. We've all experienced the frustration of someone else making noise, oblivious to how this is affecting us. So you need to work out who is sensitive to sound and who thrives with lots of noise. You may be surprised; this is not simply a case of being an outgoing and

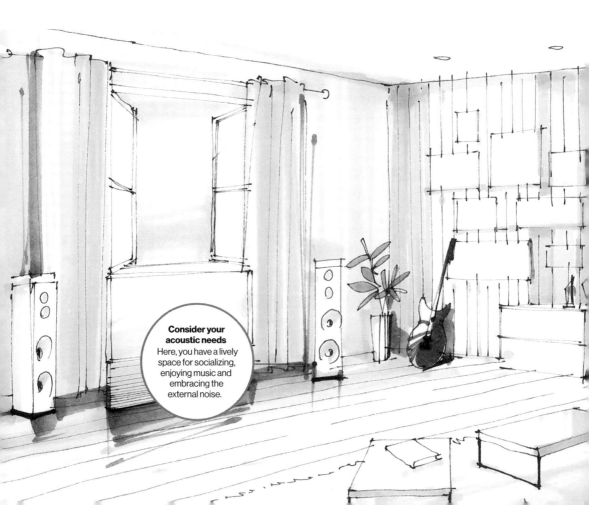

Consider your acoustic needs
Here, you have a lively space for socializing, enjoying music and embracing the external noise.

sociable person and therefore having a high threshold for noise – you can be an extrovert and get tired out in lively, noisy spaces. It may mean that you need to find some quiet time during the day to restore your energy levels and focus. On the contrary, you may find the sound of silence maddening and crave noise as a backdrop, even if you love spending time on your own.

The tip here is to recognize that these differences exist and get to know the auditory threshold of each household member, so that you can create acoustic environments to suit everyone. The following sections look at what we should be keeping an eye (or ear) out for.

You need to work out who is sensitive to sound and who thrives with lots of noise.

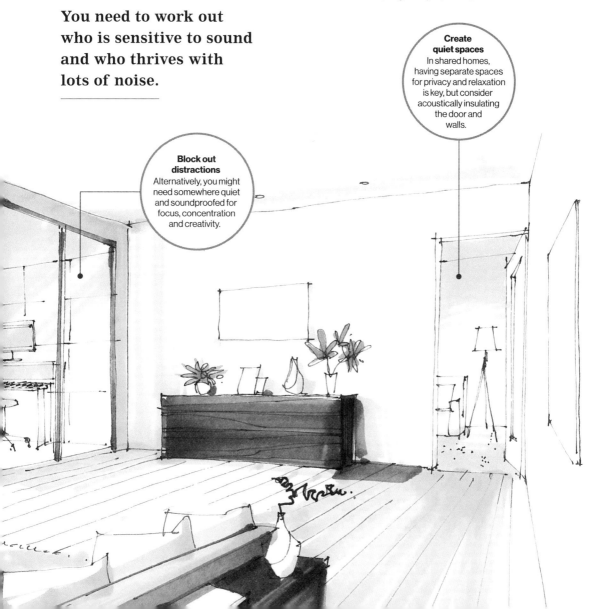

Create quiet spaces
In shared homes, having separate spaces for privacy and relaxation is key, but consider acoustically insulating the door and walls.

Block out distractions
Alternatively, you might need somewhere quiet and soundproofed for focus, concentration and creativity.

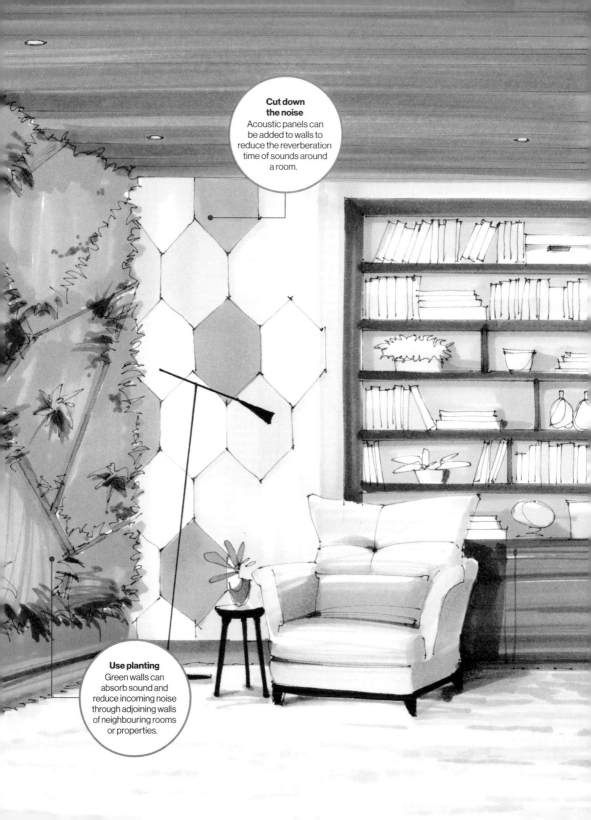

Cut down the noise
Acoustic panels can be added to walls to reduce the reverberation time of sounds around a room.

Use planting
Green walls can absorb sound and reduce incoming noise through adjoining walls of neighbouring rooms or properties.

51 | Reduce incoming noise

Public complaints about noise have increased over the last decade. In fact, 80 million Europeans live with urban noise pollution at an unacceptable level, and 40% are exposed to levels higher than 55dB at night. This is enough to raise blood pressure and increase rates of heart disease.

Consistent exposure to loud noise causes psychological and physical stress. Our homes should be peaceful sanctuaries that provide us with plenty of opportunity to recuperate and unwind. Let's look at some ways to help soundproof your home and dampen any noise disturbances that could stop you from relaxing or getting a good night's sleep.

Soundproofing can be a complex business, so let's get back to basics and explain how noise travels into our homes in the first place. Put simply, sound is the energy made when something vibrates. This energy travels via sound waves that cause objects in their path to vibrate at the same frequency. You will find some objects reduce noise more than others, which explains why simply closing your windows may not block out the road noise outside your home. Soundproofing is the process of placing obstacles in the sound waves' path that weaken its vibrations and dampen the noise. Add enough obstacles and the sound will be inaudible.

First, mend any cracks or holes in your ceilings and walls, paying particular attention to the space around vents and window frames. Inspect your doors to ensure they are sealed efficiently; consider using the draught-reducing solutions on page 137. These will help stop noise leaking through small gaps, as well as preventing energy wastage.

Larger investments would be to replace your windows with double- or triple-paned glazing, as this can dramatically reduce the sound entering your home. Or you could add layers of sound-absorbing materials to the construction of your home, such as insulating foam or fibrous material, which can both retain warmth and reduce noise transmission. To ensure these tasks are undertaken properly, they are often best installed by experienced professionals.

If you are in a rented property or on a tight budget, you could invest in a thick rug to cover hardwood floorboards or hang second-hand heavyweight curtains over leaky windows. If you have noisy neighbours on one side of your home, consider having bedrooms and the home office away from the adjoining walls if possible. If that isn't an option, rearranging your furniture and positioning a full bookcase on the boundary wall can help absorb the noise on that side of the house.

Noise and home life
In the UK, a survey of 2,000 people found that 76% thought noise affected their home life. More than half said it deterred them from opening doors and windows. The survey also found that sleep disturbed by noise can negatively affect people's health.

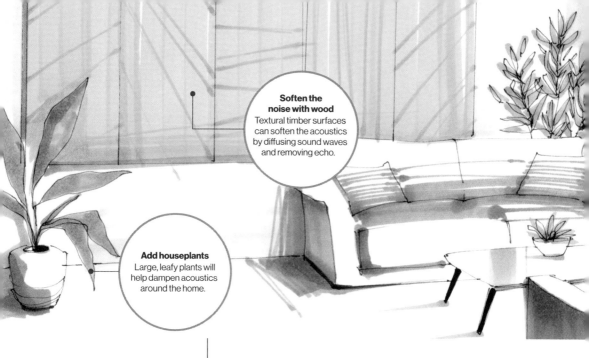

Soften the noise with wood
Textural timber surfaces can soften the acoustics by diffusing sound waves and removing echo.

Add houseplants
Large, leafy plants will help dampen acoustics around the home.

52 | Balance lively and calm acoustics

Noise created inside the home is also an issue. Excess noise has been found to be related to depression and anxiety; when it's reduced by just 5–10dB we are more relaxed, with a lower heart rate. But what can we do to control it?

First, identify the sounds. Some rooms in your home may be naturally noisier than others, which will come down to things such as how many people use the space, what they use it for and the furniture and finishes in those spaces. The kitchen, which tends to be the most sociable room in the house, is often the noisiest, with the clattering of pots and pans competing against cutlery and conversation. These sounds are amplified by the harder, wipe-clean surfaces that are common in kitchens. Hard waterproof surfaces, such as tiles on floors and walls, are often used in bathrooms, along with sinks, glass shower walls, baths, taps and mirrors.

Using more porous surfaces in these lively spaces can take the edge off the din by absorbing some of the sound. While no one wants to see the revival of carpeted kitchens and bathrooms, try introducing textiles where possible. Washable rugs, tablecloths and mats, wall hangings, towels and robes, window coverings and seat cushions can all be brought in to soften the noise in these spaces.

Rooms such as the bedroom and living room will tend to be acoustically calmer, due to the softer furniture, fabrics and furnishings that help fulfil the purpose of these spaces. If you find the acoustics are a little lively,

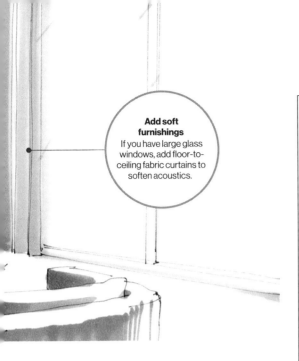

Add soft furnishings
If you have large glass windows, add floor-to-ceiling fabric curtains to soften acoustics.

HOW TO SOFTEN ACOUSTICS

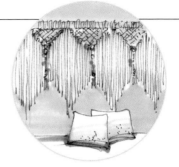

Add fabric to walls – wall hangings such as macramé or tapestries can soften otherwise-hard, reflective surfaces.

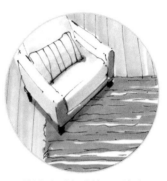

Think of soft furnishings not just from an aesthetic point of view but also as a way to improve the way a space feels by absorbing sound.

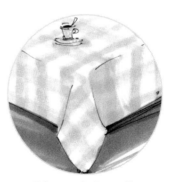

Tailor acoustics for specific activities such as using a table cloth at a dinner party to dampen noise.

consider whether you can add any more textured materials. For example, wood reflects sounds when smooth, so look for natural textured finishes with a raised grain when trying to soften the acoustics, as these can help diffuse sound waves and remove echoes. You might incorporate waney-edged wooden shelves (these have one edge left in its natural shape) or acoustic plywood panels (perforated wood with holes or grooves).

Another solution, as mentioned earlier, is to choose the right space for the right activity. If possible, keep quiet spaces for people with low acoustic thresholds away from loud areas where you might entertain, listen to music or watch surround-sound TV.

If your bedroom shares a wall with the living room, try to position furniture or wardrobes against the adjoining wall to dampen sound transmission and separate one space from the next. It may seem like common sense, but this can get overlooked in favour of aesthetics.

Finally, large, leafy plants will also help dampen acoustics around the home (see page 170 for guidance).

53 Choose quiet products

We become habituated to the acoustic soundscape of our lives, but our brains are constantly filtering out this needless input. Just think of the brain power we could save if the background noise wasn't there in the first place.

You may be familiar with the clunking boiler switching on early in the morning, or the loud spinning noise your washing machine makes – sometimes it sounds as though it's going to take off! Where possible, check the acoustic output of products before you buy – this will often be noted in product specification. This is particularly useful when choosing items that are switched on all the time, such as extractor fans or fridge-freezers, which become more

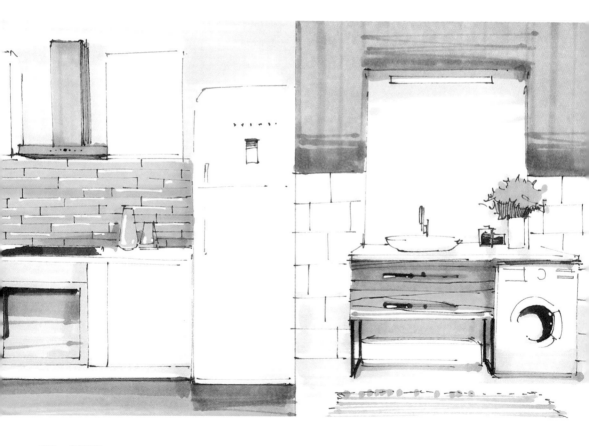

Quiet Mark is an internationally recognized award programme that assesses the noise levels of products to help consumers make an informed decision.

noticeable when the home falls quiet at bedtime. Alternatively, leave it to third-party certification and choose products and appliances with a Quiet Mark award to maintain peaceful acoustics in your home.

Quiet Mark is an internationally recognized award programme that assesses the noise levels of products to help consumers make an informed decision. Quiet Mark identifies the quietest products within each category to allow for a more serene domestic environment. You can find all these recommended products on the Quiet Mark website, from quiet kitchens to quiet gardens.

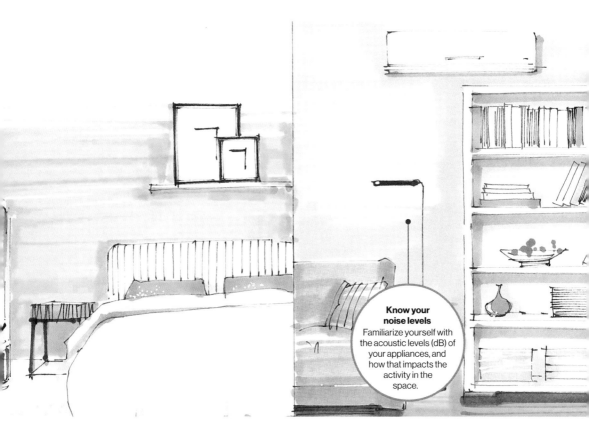

Know your noise levels
Familiarize yourself with the acoustic levels (dB) of your appliances, and how that impacts the activity in the space.

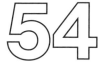# Have biophilic acoustics

If you live near a main road and are lucky enough to have a front garden or outdoor space, nature can help you create biophilic acoustics. These control the quality of sound by incorporating nature or natural elements: establishing natural sound barriers to reduce unwanted noise, or sound masking to disguise it.

Natural sound barriers can be created by growing hedges and trees, instead of building walls and fences, to mark perimeters. Increased vegetation outdoors has been found to have a significant dampening effect on noise, and subsequently reduces perceived levels of noise pollution. Not only will plants and trees absorb and disperse the sounds that would otherwise reach the windows and walls of your homes, but they'll also reduce air pollution and bring wildlife into the surrounding area.

Sound masking, by encouraging biodiversity around your home, can help disguise undesirable manmade urban noises with the sounds of nature, such as wind, water and animals. As well as planting hedges and trees, there are several ways to encourage natural sounds around your home.

You could put up bird boxes and feeders – this will encourage birds to keep returning to your garden, bringing the beneficial natural sounds of birdsong with them.

You could install wind chimes, which help you connect with the changes in weather – just make sure you like the sound they make, and that they won't disturb your neighbours! You could also install a water feature (see page 126 for more on this).

As well as sound masking, each of these can also offer non-rhythmic sensory stimuli (NRSS), catching your attention to give little beneficial moments of distraction at different times throughout the day, with restorative effects. This is called attention restoration.

Don't be disheartened if you don't have a garden. You can also use your balcony or windows to create natural sound barriers, such as hanging window boxes or trellis to grow plants vertically and create permeable green walls. You could also put up birdfeeders on your windows – just be careful you don't block out too much natural light. There may be a compromise here between letting natural light in, reducing unwanted noises and encouraging nature sounds. You will need to consider which is your priority and would work best in your home.

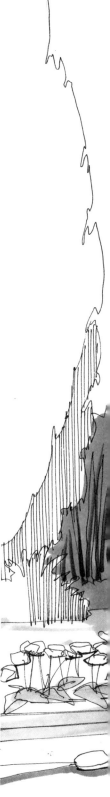

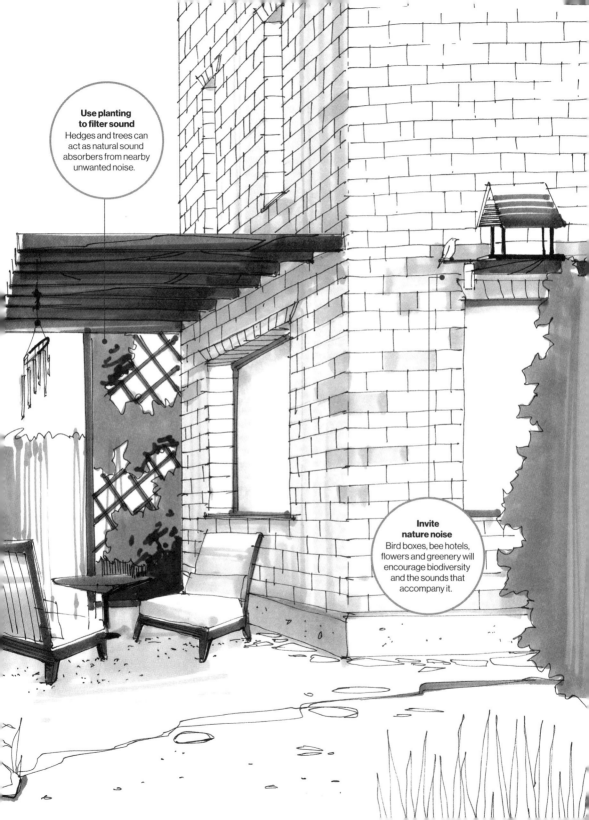

Use planting to filter sound
Hedges and trees can act as natural sound absorbers from nearby unwanted noise.

Invite nature noise
Bird boxes, bee hotels, flowers and greenery will encourage biodiversity and the sounds that accompany it.

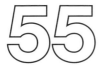

Mask unwanted noise

If you can't encourage nature sounds around your home or reduce unwanted noise, you could try using recorded nature sounds on audio devices.

These could be anything that you enjoy listening to, from birdsong or waves lapping to the sound of a forest or falling rain. Research has found that birdsong is perceived as calm, traffic as chaotic, and the sound of people as eventful. We perform best when listening to sounds we are familiar with. Think about the landscapes you have experienced and have pleasant associations with, and choose corresponding sounds for maximum benefits.

If you find nature sounds distracting, there are other options for sound masking. Noises that can reduce the difference between the background ambient hum and sudden loud sounds (such as construction work, slamming doors or shouting) include:

• **White noise** – this is a continuous mechanical-type noise, like the gentle hum of a motor, that covers the whole hearing range of frequencies. It is often used to mask background noise to aid focus and sleep, and is particularly effective for babies.

• **Pink noise** – this noise boosts lower frequencies for those who find white noise too sharp, and is more akin to natural noises such as steady rainfall or wind rustling through the leaves in a tree. Some studies are suggesting that pink noise can enhance sleep and focus.

• **Brown noise** – this is even lower frequency noise, like thunder or a crashing waterfall.

There are even apps in which you can design your own noise, changing the levels of bass, treble and mid-range sounds to suit your own preferences.

For some, music that doesn't have singing, or drum sounds, can help them focus. Research has also found that listening to high-frequency music can reduce stress. Try different types of sound to work out which ones suit you and the tasks you need to do.

NOISES FOR SOUND MASKING

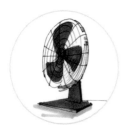

White noise is a mechanical-type noise like the gentle hum of a motor.

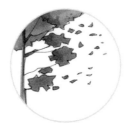

Pink noise boosts lower frequencies for those who find white noise too sharp.

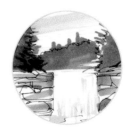

Brown noise is an even lower frequency noise, like thunder or a crashing waterfall.

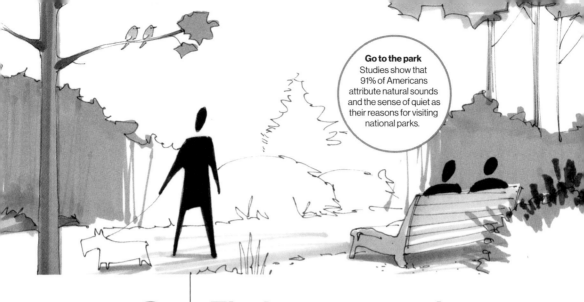

Go to the park
Studies show that 91% of Americans attribute natural sounds and the sense of quiet as their reasons for visiting national parks.

56 | Find your acoustic circadian rhythms

In urban environments, we no longer wake up with the dawn chorus and settle down for the night with the hum of crickets. But just as our circadian rhythms are affected by exposure to natural light (see pages 70–81), sounds can act as cues for our sense of time and how we feel.

You can influence your mood by playing sounds or music according to how you want to feel at a given time of day. Playing natural sound has been found to affect bodily systems that allow us to relax and our brains to rest, such as our fight-or-flight and rest-digest autonomic nervous systems. What's more, we are actually aware of this effect: natural sounds have also been found to reduce agitation and anxiety that is self-reported.

Natural sounds have been found to reduce self-reported agitation and anxiety.

There are alarm clocks that can help with your acoustic circadian rhythms by playing birdsong to wake you and the sound of waves lapping as you go to sleep. If this doesn't appeal, try creating your own soundtrack for the day. Starting the day with lively or higher frequency music and ending it with slower, calmer and more relaxing music or sounds (think resonating low hum) might help you sleep better and feel more energized.

You could also try taking a walk early in the morning and at end of the day, listening out for any nature sounds that could help you connect with the natural systems in your local environment, such as the time of day, the weather and the season. Research has found that 91% of Americans report that natural sounds and the sense of quiet motivate them to go to national parks.

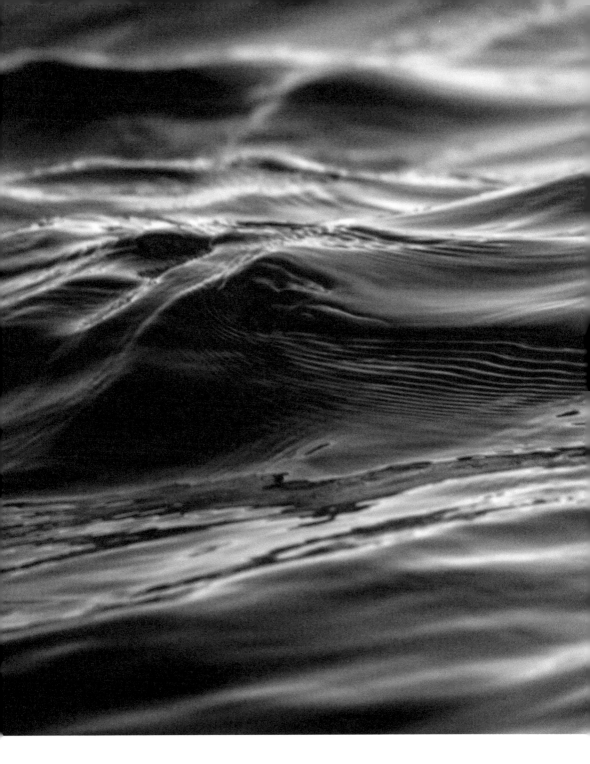

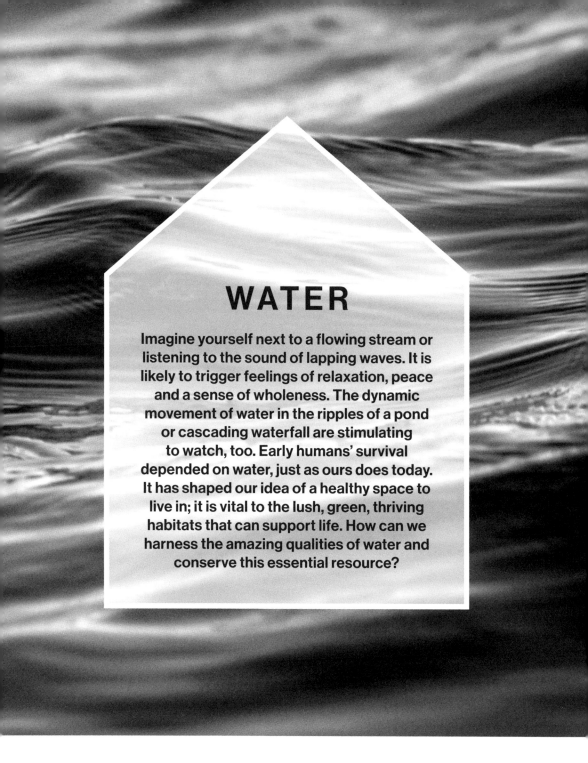

WATER

Imagine yourself next to a flowing stream or listening to the sound of lapping waves. It is likely to trigger feelings of relaxation, peace and a sense of wholeness. The dynamic movement of water in the ripples of a pond or cascading waterfall are stimulating to watch, too. Early humans' survival depended on water, just as ours does today. It has shaped our idea of a healthy space to live in; it is vital to the lush, green, thriving habitats that can support life. How can we harness the amazing qualities of water and conserve this essential resource?

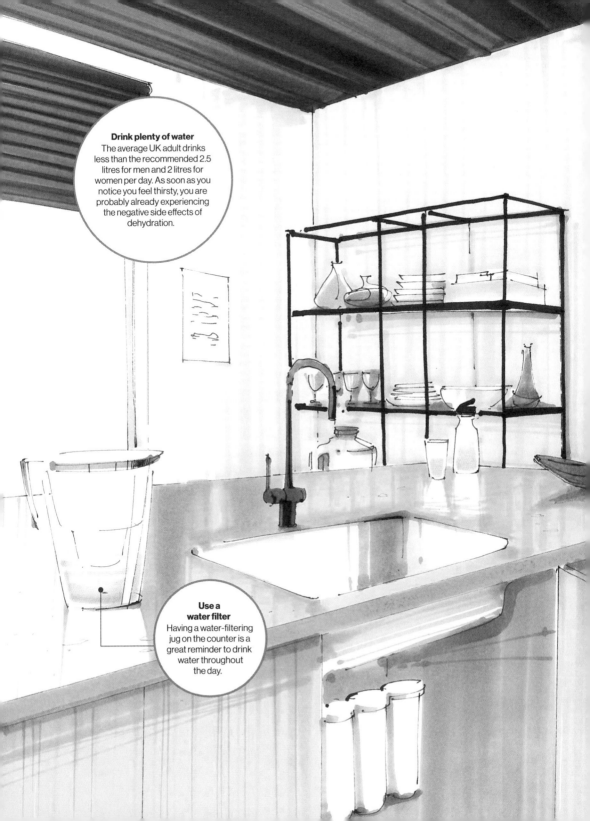

Drink plenty of water
The average UK adult drinks less than the recommended 2.5 litres for men and 2 litres for women per day. As soon as you notice you feel thirsty, you are probably already experiencing the negative side effects of dehydration.

Use a water filter
Having a water-filtering jug on the counter is a great reminder to drink water throughout the day.

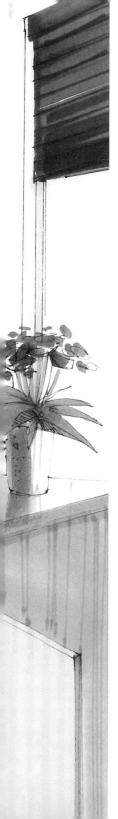

57 | Enjoy clean drinking water

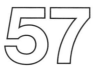

Drinking enough fresh, clean water every day is a prerequisite for health and wellbeing. Even mild levels of dehydration can lead to negative effects such as fatigue and dizziness, mood swings and headaches, increased hunger, decreased metabolism, lower reaction times and a reduction in cognitive abilities.

The most obvious and practical way to feel the benefits of water is to ensure you have easy access to clean drinking water. Although most developed countries have good water available straight from the tap, it can contain organic and inorganic contaminants, either in the water itself or from the piping and treatment systems. These include metals, minerals, chemicals, endocrine disruptors (chemicals that can affect our hormones), bacteria and viruses. We recommend filtering your drinking water in one of these ways:

• **having a range of reusable drinking bottles** to use while out, or even at home.

• **using a water filtering jug** – this is perfect for a small household or if you're renting, but filters need to be changed often (they can be recycled, but you get through a lot of them).

• **using a counter-top water filtering urn** – if you have space, this will ensure you always have plenty of filtered water for cooking and drinking, which is great for large households.

• **fitting a counter-top water filter** that is attached to your tap and draws water directly from it.

• **installing a water filtering system** under your kitchen sink – it is attached to the water pipe coming into the house so that the water coming out of the tap has already passed through the filter.

• **installing a whole-house filtration system** – this may be an option if the water is really bad where you live and you don't even want to brush your teeth with it, or you live in a hard-water area where you get a build-up of limescale in your toilet, shower head and taps (it could also save you money on maintenance and replacement pipes in the long run).

Each of these options will need filters changing regularly to reap the benefits. The cheaper systems at the top of the list will need filters changing more often than those towards the bottom. If you are concerned about water quality, it's worth getting your home supply tested.

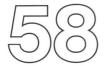

58 | Turn your bathroom into a retreat

The bathroom is one of the first places we go in the morning, and the last place we go before bed. Making a single space suitable for setting us up for the day and winding us down for sleep deserves some proper consideration. However, bathrooms are typically quite small, sometimes windowless rooms.

First, let's look at how to create a bathroom retreat for private time. Try to make this a rich, multisensory environment. Think of those magical bathrooms you see in photographs with a bathtub next to a full-wall window, immersed in a lush forest. Although we can't all achieve that, we can work out what's so appealing about that scene and then emulate it. Here are some ideas.

• **Have a soft lighting option**, such as cabinet lights, mirror lights or dimmable lighting for relaxing in the evening.

• **Bring in calming scents** using atomizers and bath oils – perhaps lavender in the evening to relax, or citrus smells in the morning to invigorate.

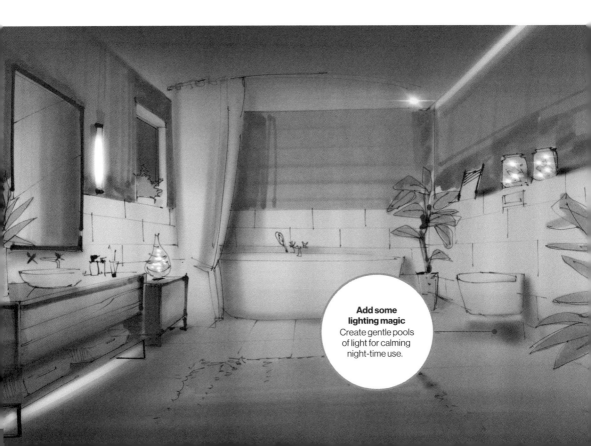

Add some lighting magic
Create gentle pools of light for calming night-time use.

- **Add a lock to your door** to add privacy.
- **Use natural, paraben-free products** that are kind to your skin – you could have soaps scented with different herbs to create different atmospheres.
- **Consider the haptic quality of soft towels**, bathmats, exfoliators and fluffy robes – a spa day doesn't feel luxurious for no reason!
- **Add some lush green plants** to the space for their recuperative benefits. In small bathrooms, plants can be hung from the ceiling or along the walls for an immersive but space-saving experience (see page 180).

When designing your bathroom retreat, try to include sensory contrasts that keep you in the moment, such as cool floor tiles and soft bathmats, warm water and exfoliating loofahs to create experiences that will enrich the time you spend there.

Lastly, if it's the restorative effects of water you're after, why not look into cold-water bathing? We don't all have access to the sea, a lake or a river, but you can make a start with a "treatment" at home. Research has found that when undertaken regularly, cold-water immersion can boost your metabolism, and cold-water showers may be more beneficial than medication for treating depression. It's chilly, but wonderful!

Try to make your bathroom a rich, multisensory environment.

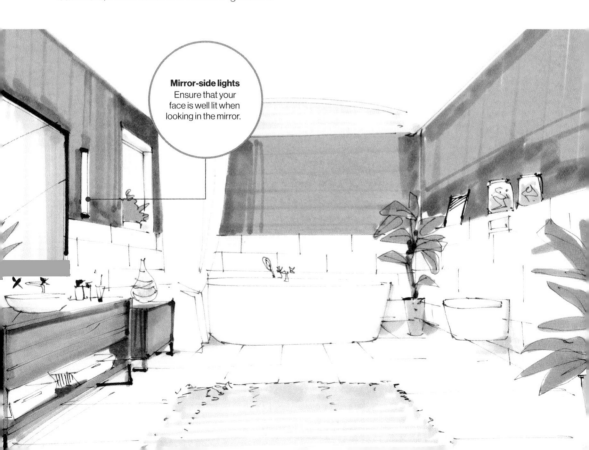

Mirror-side lights
Ensure that your face is well lit when looking in the mirror.

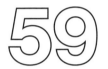

Make a shared bathroom work

While it's often good to have time alone in the bathroom, you may have no choice but to share it – and, as unlikely as this may sound, the bathroom can also be a social space.

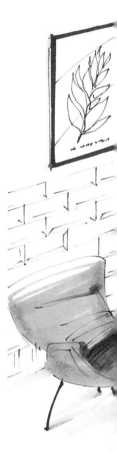

On the livelier end of the spectrum, this might be your kids' bath time, or you might be getting ready to go out with friends. For these occasions, bright lighting is important, as well as good storage for toys and beauty products to make more space and avoid too much mess. Another way to keep things organized when the bathroom gets busy is to put hooks on the back of the door for towels.

You might also like someone to join you while you have a relaxing evening bath or brush your teeth and get ready for bed; this might be one of the few opportunities you get to talk through your day with your partner. Having somewhere they can sit while you chat which is a bit comfier than the closed toilet seat is a good, and often

overlooked, consideration. You could bring in an extra chair, or a storage trunk could double up as a cushioned seat. This is a great way to make the bathroom a more intimate and inclusive space to be shared.

Think about ventilation
Operable windows and good ventilation are key for when the bathroom floor becomes swamped with damp towels and water has been splashed across the floor.

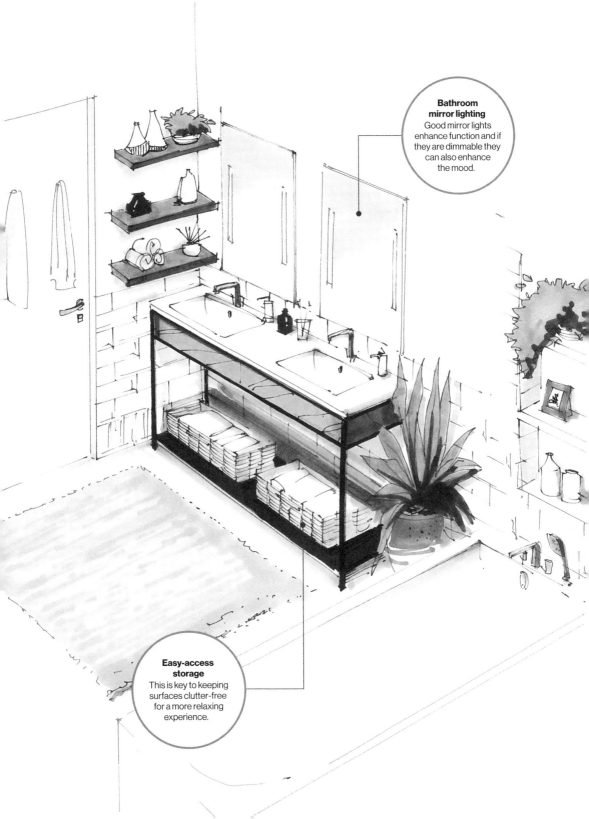

Bathroom mirror lighting
Good mirror lights enhance function and if they are dimmable they can also enhance the mood.

Easy-access storage
This is key to keeping surfaces clutter-free for a more relaxing experience.

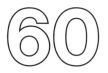 # Save water in the kitchen

Being more water efficient in your home is not only a great way to save money, which in turn will reduce your stress levels, but is also kinder to the environment. Here are a few ways you can cut down on your water usage in the kitchen.

Try using a washing-up bowl to contain warm soapy water and minimize continuous tap use. Foot pedal taps are a hands-free, foot-operated system for dispensing water, which are affordable and have many advantages over traditional hand-operated taps. Not only do they allow you to control the water supply more efficiently, but they are also very hygienic.

Picture this: you have just kneaded some dough, or dug up some muddy carrots from the garden. What's the first thing you will want to do? Wash your hands! The pedal tap allows you to turn on the water without having to touch anything, keeping your kitchen clean and tidy. This also makes it a great option for multi-taskers who are likely to be found juggling multiple utensils with their hands full!

Another way to save precious water in your kitchen is to put down the sponge and use an energy star-rated dishwasher. It's a common misconception that washing by hand uses less water; modern dishwashers use as little as 6 litres per cycle, which is about the same or even less than an average hand wash. If you run your dishwasher on a full load, you'll not only conserve water, but you'll also make the most of your washing detergent.

WATER-SAVING TIPS

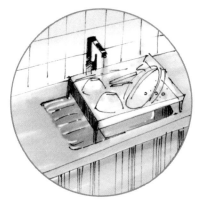

Use a washing-up bowl so that you can wash up without having the tap running.

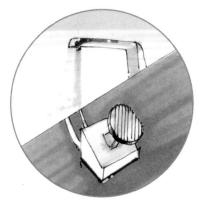

Try hands-free foot pedal taps; these allow you to control the water usage, and are also hygienic.

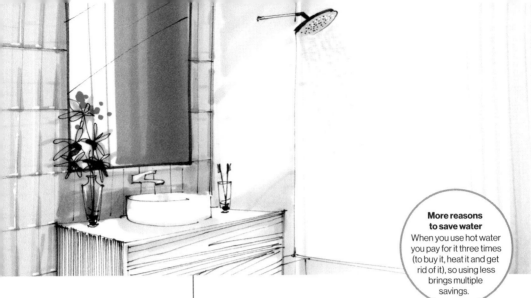

More reasons to save water
When you use hot water you pay for it three times (to buy it, heat it and get rid of it), so using less brings multiple savings.

61 | Save water in the bathroom

The bathroom is the main source of wasted water in our homes, but it is also the easiest place to conserve it: a long shower or deep bath make up around 34% of our water consumption. Here are some tips to get you started.

Did you know that a full bathtub can use up to 80 litres of water? This makes baths seem like more of a luxury. Even 3 centimetres less water in your bath can save 5 litres. You should also make sure that you fit the plug before you turn on the tap to find the right temperature.

The average shower head uses around 12 litres of water per minute, and power showers use as much as 23 litres per minute. Opt for shorter showers – 5 minutes is good, compared to the average of 10 minutes. If you tend to lose track of time in the shower, you can buy a timer as a reminder. Even better, invest in a low-flow, water-restricting or aerating shower head, which can use 60% less water than a standard shower head. Aerating taps on sinks are also an option and can reduce the water flow by 50%. They can be easy to replace, and you'll start saving as soon as you use them.

Small habits like remembering to turn the tap off while brushing your teeth or shaving can really help; otherwise, it really is water down the drain. Even a leaky tap can waste up to 25 litres of water per day – just imagine all those bottles lined up! It can be fixed in minutes and very cheaply with a new washer.

Lastly, in our crazy, inefficient world, a standard toilet will flush 13 litres of drinking-quality water down the drain, which accounts for 30% of our water use. Fitting a dual-flush cistern can be more water efficient, only using between 2.6 and 4 litres. These systems can be prone to leakages, so look out for water draining into the bowl of your WC and fix leaky washers if that occurs. There are also grey water systems that divert waste water from showers and basins to your WC, but these are surprisingly expensive and complicated to fit, often making the cost prohibitive.

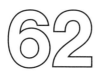

Consider installing
a home aquarium

We often bring objects into our homes that remind us of positive experiences we've had with water. This could be an evocative painting of a seascape, gentle fabric patterns that imitate water ripples, or pebbles, shells and driftwood collected from the seaside. All of these objects remind us of pleasurable experiences we've had, and in turn make us feel good. To take this a step further, you could create a blue space in your home.

The most common water features we see in people's homes are aquariums, and if you need help winding down after a long day, a fish tank could be a great addition to your home. Watching the movement of the fish before going to sleep can help you relax and unwind, while the sounds the tank makes can help mask unwanted noise when drifting off. You could also consider placing a fish tank in your study, as the gentle movement and ripples of water reflecting light is a good form of non-rhythmic sensory stimuli (NRSS; see page 43), which can help restore attention and improve focus.

Aquariums also offer an opportunity for people with busy lifestyles or allergies to have a pet. However, home aquariums do need regular maintenance to ensure your fish friends are well cared for. Make sure you commit to a regular feeding schedule and change the water weekly.

Fish tanks in waiting rooms

Have you ever wondered why doctors' and dentists' waiting rooms so often have fish tanks in them? Research has found that spending time by a fish tank can lower heart rate and blood pressure, and that their hypnotic quality can reduce pain.

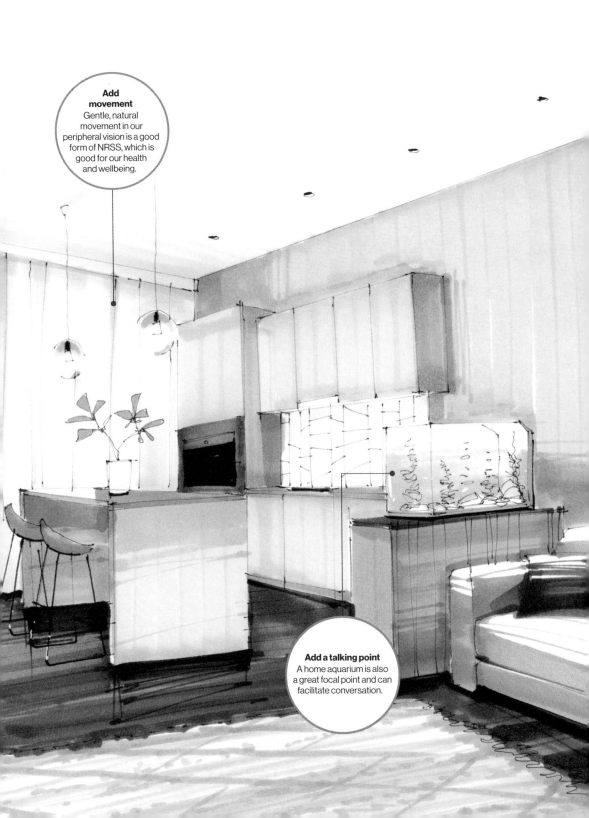

Add movement
Gentle, natural movement in our peripheral vision is a good form of NRSS, which is good for our health and wellbeing.

Add a talking point
A home aquarium is also a great focal point and can facilitate conversation.

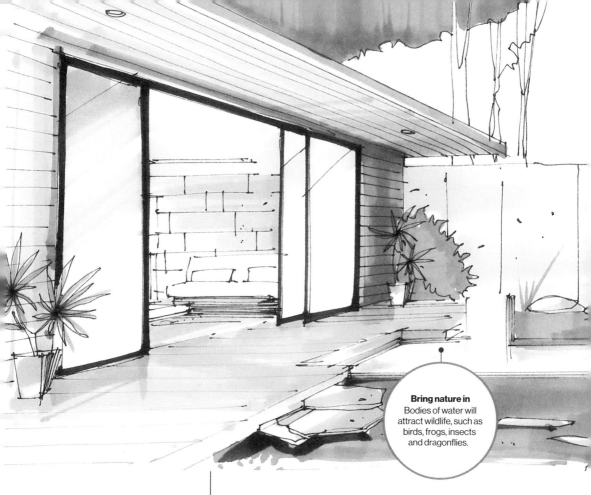

Bring nature in
Bodies of water will attract wildlife, such as birds, frogs, insects and dragonflies.

63 | Install a garden water feature

The introduction of a water feature into your garden brings many benefits. It can serve as a focal point, attract wildlife, reduce stress levels and enhance your overall experience of your garden. Here are a few points to consider.

We tend to gravitate towards blue spaces because we find the presence of water inherently soothing, so you might consider placing a garden water feature where you want people to gather. This may be on the patio or decking area, or elsewhere near some seating. Think about incorporating lighting with your water feature, as this will enhance the visual quality of the water's movement. If you can, position the water feature in such a way that it bounces reflections of sunlight onto the ceiling of your home. That way, you

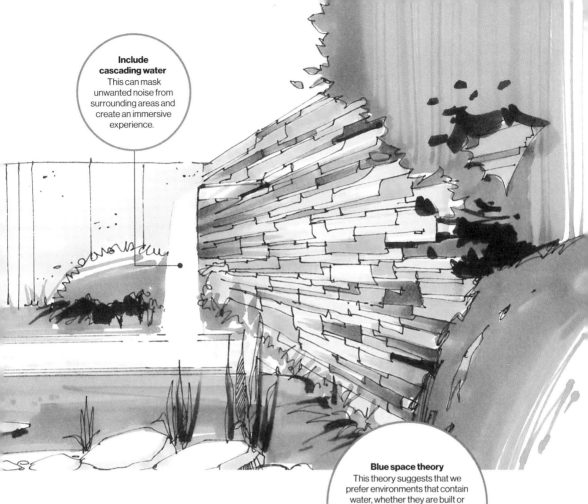

Include cascading water
This can mask unwanted noise from surrounding areas and create an immersive experience.

Blue space theory
This theory suggests that we prefer environments that contain water, whether they are built or natural. They have a positive effect on us, feeling more restorative than spaces without water in them.

will benefit from its presence both when you are inside and outside.

Water features can come in all different styles, enriching both modern and traditional gardens. You could choose a classic lily pond or an ornate birdbath for an older property, or a water sculpture with clean lines that would suit a more modern garden. When deciding which type of water feature to go for, consider if you want to incorporate a fountain or mini water cascade to help mask unwanted background noise that may be coming from a loud nearby road or noisy neighbours.

Bird baths, and ponds in particular, are a great way to attract wildlife into your garden and increase biodiversity. Over the last 100 years, around 70% of ponds in Britain are thought to have disappeared, yet ponds attract a whole menagerie of creatures, including dragonflies, birds, frogs and insects. They also offer us the opportunity to connect with natural systems such as the seasons and weather, as the pond life will change from month to month.

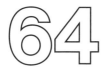

Use rainwater for plants

As populations grow and climate change causes the earth's temperatures to rise, an increasing amount of pressure is being put on our water supplies. Throughout the hot, dry summer months, water resources become more valuable than ever. Young plants are particularly vulnerable during these seasons as they need extra watering while they get rooted in the soil and find the moisture layers deep below. Catching and storing rainwater is a cheap, easy solution to meet your plants' needs without having to turn on the main tap so frequently.

Any structure that has a gutter and a down pipe can collect rainwater. This could be the roof of your home, your garden shed or even your greenhouse. All you need to do is invest in a water butt system with a diverter. Make sure you position your water butt on even ground, so it doesn't topple over when it fills up. It's also advisable to use a lid to stop any wildlife falling in, and avoid attracting mosquitoes.

Once installed, the water butt collects the rainwater from the down pipe and is designed to allow any overflow to run back into the drain.

Your plants will love being watered with rainwater because it isn't treated with chemicals like the water from a hose.

Make sure you give your water butt an annual clean to avoid the build-up of any nasties, and if you have several water butts, consider rotating which one you draw water from. This will ensure you always use the freshest water supply.

Benefit your plants
Young plants are particularly vulnerable during the hot summer months and will love their chemical-free showers.

Your plants will love being watered with rainwater because it isn't treated with chemicals, like the water from a hose.

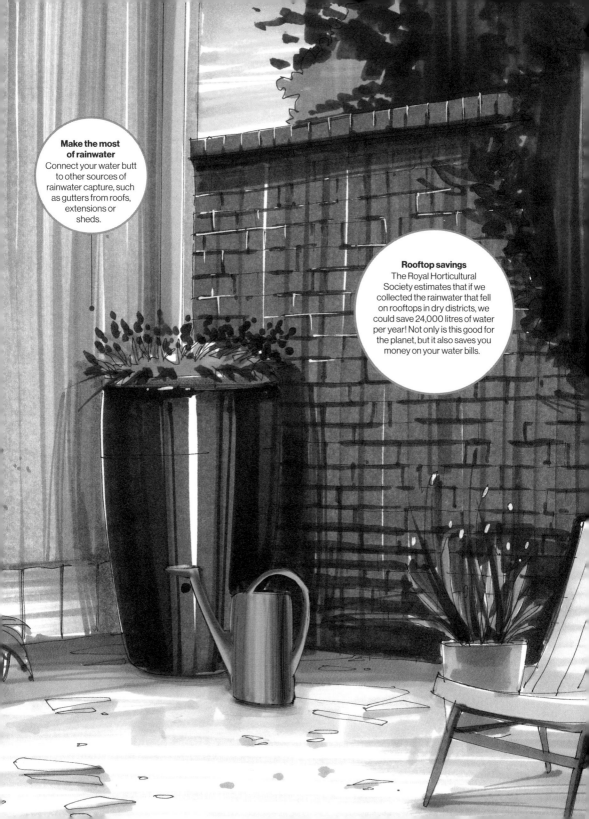

Make the most of rainwater
Connect your water butt to other sources of rainwater capture, such as gutters from roofs, extensions or sheds.

Rooftop savings
The Royal Horticultural Society estimates that if we collected the rainwater that fell on rooftops in dry districts, we could save 24,000 litres of water per year! Not only is this good for the planet, but it also saves you money on your water bills.

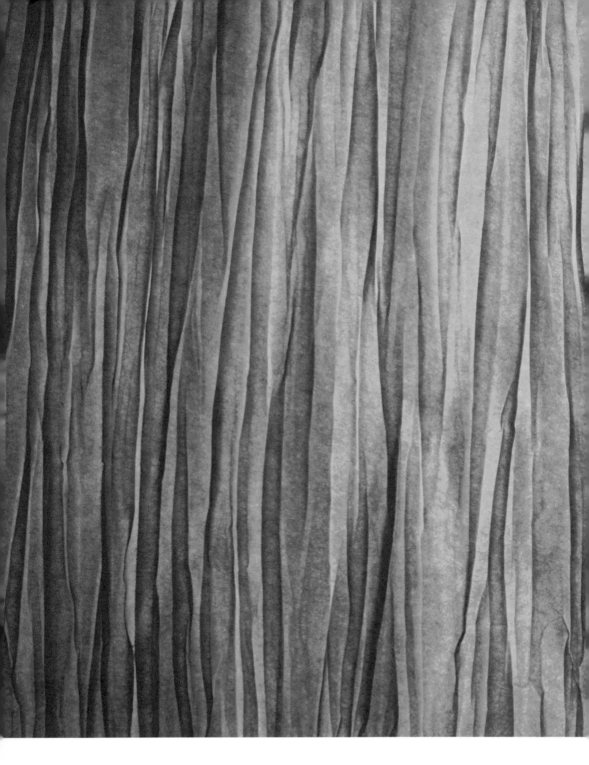

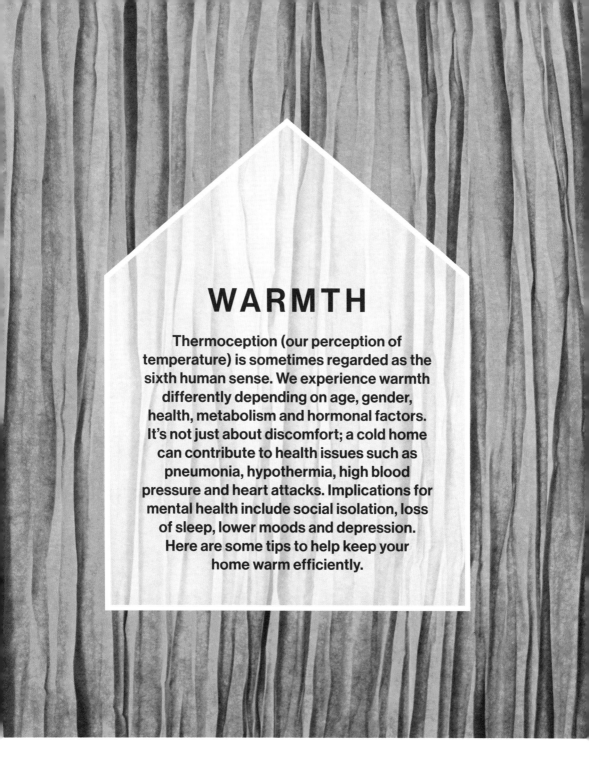

WARMTH

Thermoception (our perception of temperature) is sometimes regarded as the sixth human sense. We experience warmth differently depending on age, gender, health, metabolism and hormonal factors. It's not just about discomfort; a cold home can contribute to health issues such as pneumonia, hypothermia, high blood pressure and heart attacks. Implications for mental health include social isolation, loss of sleep, lower moods and depression. Here are some tips to help keep your home warm efficiently.

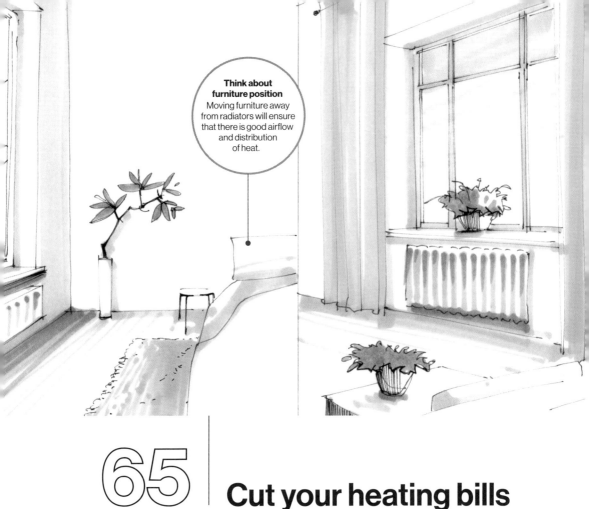

Think about furniture position
Moving furniture away from radiators will ensure that there is good airflow and distribution of heat.

65 | Cut your heating bills

Heating your home can be a stressful business. Not only is it expensive, but it can also be the biggest contributor to your carbon footprint levels. Here are some ways to stay warm, keep heating costs down and reduce your stress levels when the bills come in, all of which will improve your wellbeing.

The simplest things to do before turning up the thermostat are to throw on a jumper, get yourself some thick, cosy socks or grab a hot water bottle for the night. You might also want to consider switching energy providers to get a better deal. In the UK, this could mean a saving of around £300 per year. Look for companies that supply renewable energy so you can do your bit for the environment –

these are no longer the most expensive options, so it is worth shopping around.

Another simple solution is to ensure you have good airflow around radiators to allow convection currents to distribute the heat, by positioning your furniture further away from your radiator. If your favourite sofa or armchair sits directly in front of your radiator, it will absorb most of the heat and prevent the hot

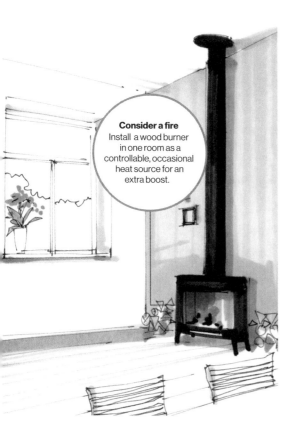

Consider a fire
Install a wood burner in one room as a controllable, occasional heat source for an extra boost.

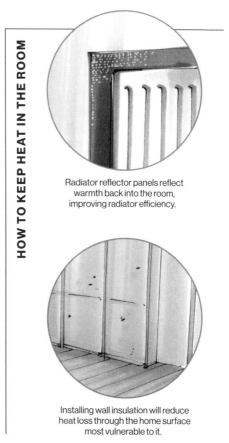

Radiator reflector panels reflect warmth back into the room, improving radiator efficiency.

Installing wall insulation will reduce heat loss through the home surface most vulnerable to it.

air from circulating freely around the room.

You can also fit radiator reflector panels that reflect hot air back into the room to boost circulation even more. You can find them at general hardware stores, and they are easy to install, and a great way to make the best use of your precious heat.

Get your boiler and radiators serviced regularly to keep them running efficiently and safely. This can also help remove air build-up in radiators, which can prevent them from warming up.

Find out about getting your home fully insulated (consider floors, walls and roof spaces) – it's remarkable what a difference it will make, especially when you consider that the average home's heat loss is 35% through walls, 25% through roofs and 15% through floors. Each of these areas needs a different approach to insulation, and this will depend on

Position furniture away from radiators to allow hot air to circulate.

the construction type of your home. As there are numerous technical and practical issues, it is best to get an expert in to discuss the best approach and quote for what is possible (grants are often available to help you do this). Insulating your home is easier than you'd think, and the sooner you get it done the sooner you will save money and keep your home warm.

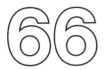

66 | Ditch your dryer

We've come to rely on technology. But the reality is, we don't always need it. If we can harness what we already have, we might realize that dryers aren't essential at all: perhaps it's one fewer item that we have to buy and maintain.

The annual power use per person for tumble dryers is three times greater than for washing machines. So a good way to reduce your energy bills, and make the most of the warmth already in your home, is to ditch your noisy, electricity-guzzling dryer and opt for a smart way to air-dry your clothes. In a utility room,

or a convenient space near a radiator, fit a suspended drying rail to the ceiling joists. You can hang your washing and leave it to dry overnight in the warm air that rises towards the ceiling, and that you're already paying for.

However, mechanical ventilation, such as a continuous running fan, is essential for this tip

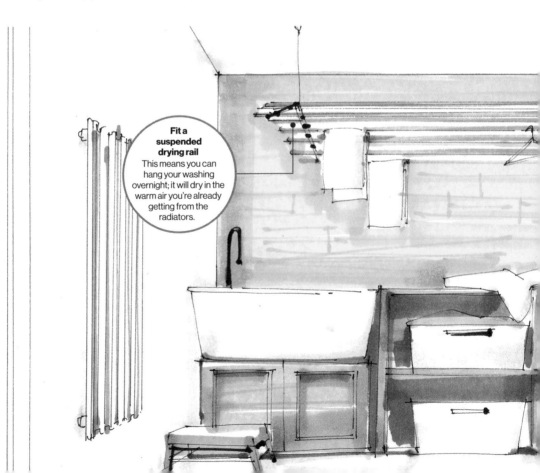

Fit a suspended drying rail
This means you can hang your washing overnight; it will dry in the warm air you're already getting from the radiators.

to work: the possible associated health issues caused by insufficient ventilation in the home (see pages 144–5) will outweigh any benefits to energy consumption.

A study conducted by the Mackintosh Environmental Architecture research unit in Scotland found that 87% of people dried their clothes passively indoors and 64% did this on or near sources of heat. This causes a problem: many households have moisture levels above the upper threshold for dust-mite growth, and problems with damp and mould. The study concluded that drying space should be separate from the rest of the house and should have its own designated heat and ventilation. This will enable the warm, dry air to be drawn up over the clothes and sucked out from above, along with any moisture.

Most continuous running fans will run much more quietly and more energy-efficiently than traditional timer-controlled extractor fans. This is an energy saving solution – just make sure you do it right, with proper ventilation to keep your home healthy.

Mechanical ventilation, is essential for air-drying to work, in order to avoid health issues associated with insufficient ventilation.

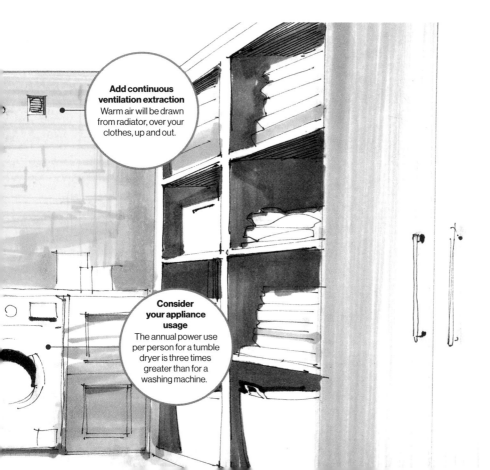

Add continuous ventilation extraction
Warm air will be drawn from radiator, over your clothes, up and out.

Consider your appliance usage
The annual power use per person for a tumble dryer is three times greater than for a washing machine.

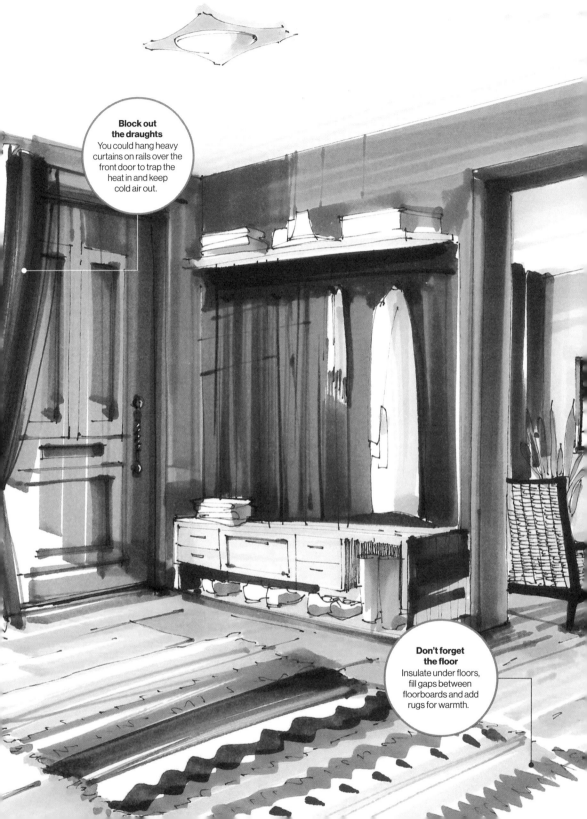

Block out the draughts
You could hang heavy curtains on rails over the front door to trap the heat in and keep cold air out.

Don't forget the floor
Insulate under floors, fill gaps between floorboards and add rugs for warmth.

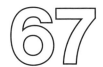

Consider a stove
Replace your open fireplace with an enclosed log-burning stove to prevent chimney draughts.

67 | Diminish the draughts

Draughts occur when gaps or openings allow air to enter or escape your home, making it chilly in the winter months. They differ from ventilation as they are unplanned and can happen anywhere, rather than in the places where you want a good air flow, such as in bathrooms, kitchens, WCs and utility spaces.

When it comes to keeping cold air out, draught proofing is an effective option and can save you 10% on your annual heating bill. Here are the most common causes of draughts, and what to do about them:

• **Internal doors** – investigate whether there are any gaps around the edges; check if you can see through to the other side of the door, then, on a cold day, hold your hand over different parts of the door, all around the edges and at the bottom. If you can see a gap, or feel cold air, fit wiper strips or a brush seal to prevent air escaping. You could also hang heavy curtains on rails over the doors to trap the heat in and invest in

(or make your own) draught excluders. Draught excluders are cost effective and flexible, and can be stored away during the warmer months. Remember to focus on draught-proofing the doors to the outside, as well as those that lead to rooms you don't heat; don't worry about the doors in between two heated rooms, as the warm air can freely circulate here.

• **Front doors** – extra measures you can take here include fitting an escutcheon cover over the keyhole, installing a letterbox flap or brush and making sure your letter box fixings are well oiled, so the flap doesn't get stuck and let warm air escape. If heat loss

Draught proofing is an effective option that can save you 10% on your annual heating bill.

through your front door is significant, consider installing an inner door or building a porch with its own door. This way, when you leave your home in the chilly months, the second door will block out gusts of cold air and stop them entering your home.

• **Windows** – a clever way to locate where a draught is coming in through your window is by moving a candle around the frame. Wherever the flame flickers, mark the spot so that you can seal it later on using weathering strips. Choose long-lasting metal ones with brushes or, if you're on a budget, self-adhesive foam strips, which are also easier to install.

Hanging curtains creates a barrier between the cold air and your cosy room. Choose full-length, thermally lined, heavyweight fabrics such as velvet or tweed, as they are tightly woven and ideal insulators. Additionally, you could hang two sets of curtains over a blind – the layering effect traps air between the materials for even better insulation. If you hang a thinner curtain first, in warmer weather you can keep the thicker curtains pulled back or take them down.

Window-shrink films are a cost-effective option. Quick and easy to install, these provide an airtight lining that can drastically improve your windows' performance. However, they will prevent you opening the window to let fresh air in, so you'll need to find alternative ways of ventilating the space to prevent damp and stale air.

If you have single-glazed windows, consider whether double or triple glazing is an option. With sash windows, perhaps they could be refurbished with draught-proofing brushes or secondary glazing installed inside the frames.

Why warmth matters
Temperature is thought to be one of the leading factors in people's dissatisfaction about the buildings in which they live and work.

If your windows have locks, make sure you tighten them fully when it's cold out. This is an easy thing to forget but can make a real difference.

• **Chimneys** – these are designed to draw warm air out of the home and continue to do so even when not in use! Luckily, there are a number of ways to draught-proof them for different budgets:

Block them when not in use with a removable chimney balloon or similar draught-excluding device (remember to remove them and have your chimney swept before using the fireplace again).

Hire a professional to fit a chimney pot cover.

Replace your open fire with a log-burning stove; these have a register plate that the stove's flue attaches to, which encloses them and prevents warm air from being drawn out of your home. This will need to be professionally fitted and meet building regulations.

• **Loft hatches** – as hot air rises in our homes, these can let warm air leak into a ventilated attic space, so consider fitting an insulated loft hatch and draught sealing around the frame.

• **Floorboards and skirting boards** – apply a filler to block any gaps, remembering that timber floorboards are prone to contracting and expanding, so make sure you purchase a product that can withstand movements to prevent cracking.

• **Old extractor fans** – have a look for any that are not in use, as these may need to be filled with brickwork or concrete. Be careful not to block off any in-use ventilation systems.

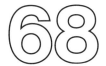

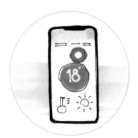

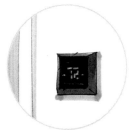

68 | Control your heating

Controlling the temperature and timing of your heating and hot water is key to managing your home's warmth and comfort, as well as saving carbon emissions and money. There are a number of ways technology can help, depending on your needs and your lifestyle.

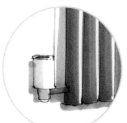

What temperature should the home be?
Preferably between 18 and 23°C and well ventilated. The exact temperature will depend on who is in the house, their age, personal preferences and activity levels. All of these may, of course, vary throughout the day.

- **Boiler** – this is likely to have controls allowing you to manage the temperature and times for your heating and hot water. Set it for when you need it, such as just mornings and evenings if you work elsewhere during the day. Bear in mind that the higher the hot water temperature, the faster your home will heat up.
- **Smart heating controls** – these allow you to control the temperature and timings of your heating system remotely, using an app. This is useful if your daily schedules change, as you can adjust your heating on the move. Some will even learn your living patterns and adjust themselves automatically, which can come in handy if you don't find it too invasive.
- **Thermostats** – these work by turning the heating on when the air temperature drops below your chosen level. Older homes often have one thermostat located in a hallway, which controls the temperature of the whole house. Although this is convenient for adjusting the dial, it can unnecessarily activate the heating for the whole house if cold air blows in. Modern homes are likely to have individual room thermostats to control the temperature in each space, which is perfect if you like your bedroom cooler than your living room.
- **Thermostatic radiator valves** – these control the flow of hot water to your radiators and allow you to control temperatures in each room, for example in a spare bedroom that doesn't need to be heated all the time. They are cost effective to buy and fairly easy to fit to existing radiators. Expensive models often have built-in timers, which can even be Wi-Fi or app controlled.
- **Boiler thermostats** – these allow you to control your water temperature if your hot water comes from a storage tank, thus avoiding scalding water or energy wastage. Adjust the dial to the desired temperature, which turns off the water-heating element when that temperature is reached.

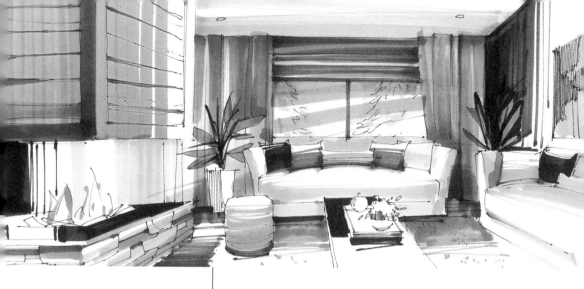

⑥⑨ | Create a cosy fireplace

Nothing beats the atmosphere a real fire brings to your home, with its dancing flames, crackling sounds and delicious smoky aroma. An open fireplace or a wood-burning stove can add so much life to a room, but which one is best suited to your space?

An open fireplace can act as a real focal point. If you have a traditional home full of character and traditional features, an open fireplace with a beautiful statement mantelpiece can serve as the centre of the home that draws people in, which is perfect for bringing friends and families together. However, an open fire is a messy and inefficient way to heat your home; 80% of the warm air is drawn up and out of the chimney and only 20% of it flows into the room.

If there is no existing fireplace, or you have less space, a wood-burning stove might be a good option, as it needs only fireproof surrounds to nearby walls. Because of this, stoves can fit very nicely in kitchens, breakfast rooms, living rooms and dining rooms, providing additional warmth and ambience.

Wood-burning stoves are also much more energy efficient, as they deliver constant heat typically at 80% efficiency (only 20% goes up the flue), saving you fuel costs.

Another factor to consider is that wood-burning stoves are much safer, as you can enclose the fire, allowing spitting sparks to be caught behind the heat-resistant glass. This means young children need less supervision around them – although caution should still be taken, as they do get extremely hot without showing it visibly.

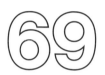

Fires and indoor air quality
All fires create PM 2.5 particles through combustion, which can pollute the atmosphere, causing respiratory and cardiovascular problems. Even more efficient wood-burning stoves contribute to this.

70 | Manage solar gain

Harnessing the power of the sun to fuel our homes is a source of green energy and comes with many benefits. However, homes must be adapted to make use of it, and manage the changing seasons and rise in temperatures.

Solar gain is the process by which our homes heat up through the sun's radiation. The heat is absorbed into the space, leaving it feeling very warm and sometimes uncomfortable. If your room faces the sun and becomes too hot in summer months, consider fitting shutters, awnings or a brise soleil to the exterior façade to provide shade – these are solutions commonly used in hotter climates. You could also consider closing your blinds or curtains during the day to block out unwanted sun rays. Planting deciduous trees outside your window will also provide you with shade in the summer, but allow the weaker winter sunshine to warm your home in the cooler months.

In the UK, windows are usually designed to retain the winter heat. This can be problematic in the summer when heat struggles to escape. However, traditional sash windows can manage the movement of hot air throughout the house, as they provide a natural, intelligent method of ventilation. When the bottom sash is raised and the top lowered, the bottom opening allows cool, fresh air to be drawn in from the outside, which then drops to the floor and pushes the hot air higher and out of the top opening. Clever!

You may be able to use this simple stack ventilation system idea to keep the whole home cooler in the summer. Try opening windows and doors on the lower floor to draw in cool air, while opening windows on upper floors to draw the warm air up and out. This system works even better if you have roof lights to open on upper floors.

Try a simple stack ventilation system to keep the house cool in summer.

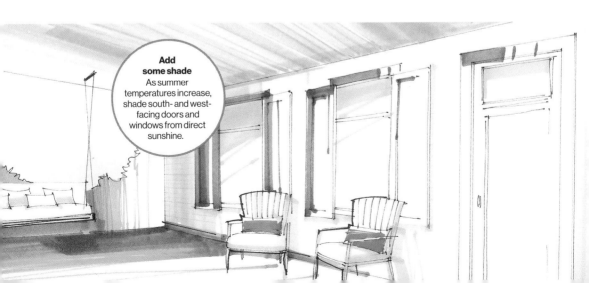

Add some shade
As summer temperatures increase, shade south- and west-facing doors and windows from direct sunshine.

AIR

As modern buildings become more sealed than ever, and we bring in more toxic man-made materials, indoor air quality has decreased. In the home, air quality is something we rarely consider; many toxins are odourless, so it often gets overlooked. We breathe 11,000 litres of air each day, so it really is something we should pay attention to, and although we can't control outdoor air pollution, we can improve air quality in the home. Here are some tips to help keep the air you and your loved ones breathe as clean and healthy as possible.

71 | Be an air-quality detective

When we think about air pollutants, we imagine traffic-choked motorways and smog-filled cities, rather than the air quality in the buildings where we spend most of our time. However, many of the tasks we do there, such as cooking, cleaning and decorating, can cause poor air quality and lead to serious health issues.

Pollution levels indoors can reach up to 100 times higher than outdoor pollution levels, and the World Health Organization has identified indoor and outdoor air pollution as the world's biggest environmental health risk. But how can you tell if the air quality in your home is at a healthy level?

The first and simplest thing to do is to trust your sense of smell. Often, you can tell if the air smells stale and notice the scent of things like exhaust fumes from passing cars, or cooking gas. However, there are many indoor air pollutants you won't be able to detect. We quickly become habituated to the smell of our own homes and, as a result, find it harder to detect recurring scents; you've probably noticed how everyone else's home has a distinct smell, yet it's hard to identify your own.

Second, be aware of symptoms caused by common air pollutants in the home. While the most shocking data about effects on health is recorded in the developing world, where exposure to smoke from cooking fires is higher, it is still important for us to consider these:

• **Carbon monoxide** – this is created through the combustion of fuels such as gas or wood, and most people

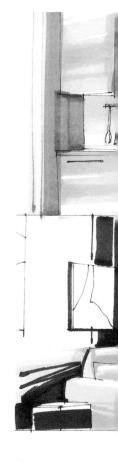

are aware of the deadly effects of breathing it in. Carbon monoxide detectors should be fitted in all houses as standard practice. However, these may not pick up some of the lower levels of carbon monoxide that stoves and fires can give off. While breathing in smaller amounts won't be as detrimental, it can still cause confusion and memory loss.

• **Fine particulate matter (PM 2.5 and PM 10)** – these small particles come from things like candles, cooking, fireplaces and smoking in the home, or from outside, due to vehicle exhausts or industrial emissions. They can create allergy-like symptoms and shortness of breath.

• **VOCs (volatile organic compounds)** – these are frequently occurring gases emitted from many materials in your home, such as paints, varnishes, cleaning products and cosmetics, as well as building materials, furniture and fabrics. Short-term effects are nausea, fatigue and throat irritation, whereas long-term VOC exposure has been linked to more serious respiratory system irritation and kidney and liver damage.

• **Radon** – this naturally occurring gas is present inside and outside. It can

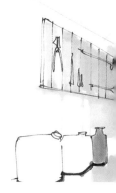

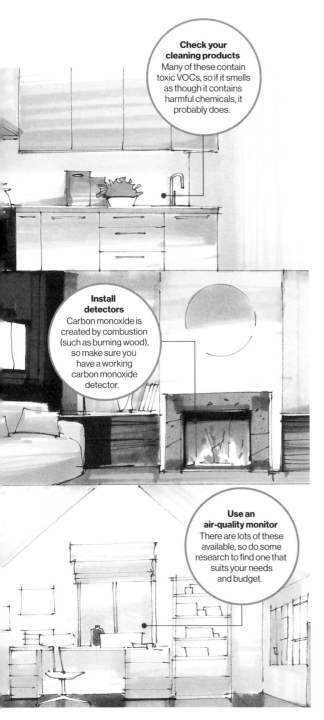

Check your cleaning products
Many of these contain toxic VOCs, so if it smells as though it contains harmful chemicals, it probably does.

Install detectors
Carbon monoxide is created by combustion (such as burning wood), so make sure you have a working carbon monoxide detector.

Use an air-quality monitor
There are lots of these available, so do some research to find one that suits your needs and budget.

cause shortness of breath, coughing, tightness in the chest, hoarseness and trouble swallowing. It is also the second most common cause of lung cancer after smoking. Radon isn't an issue in all areas, so check radon maps to see if it is prevalent near your home.

• **Carbon dioxide** – people are the main source of this, and poor ventilation. Even low concentrations (1,000ppm) can affect our cognitive function and ability to make decisions.

• **Brominated fire retardants** – these are chemicals used to reduce flammability of many products in the home, including electricals, textiles and furniture (the latter a throwback to when more people smoked in the home). They can affect hormones and neurodevelopment (developing neurological pathways to allow for normal brain function).

• **Temperature and humidity** – heating and poor ventilation are the main culprits here. At the wrong levels, they can lead to eye irritation, skin rashes and, in extreme cases, asthma attacks. Excess damp and lack of ventilation can create the perfect conditions for mould to grow.

A third option, which is becoming increasingly popular, is to use an air-quality monitor. There are many domestic devices available, but at the time of writing none of them measure all of the most common air pollutants. However, it is worth considering your priorities and which toxins you want to find out about, then researching the best option for your budget.

If you don't want to invest in this technology, the rest of the chapter explains plenty of things you can do to improve the air quality in your home.

72 Know your local air quality

We open our windows in the hope that an inflow of clean air will help flush pollutants out of our homes, but your distance from the road or other contaminating sources can have a large impact on the air in your home. Studies suggest that living 50 metres away from a road can halve the air pollution levels; while pollution caused by vehicles isn't even detectable once you get 200–300 metres away, or higher than the fifth or sixth floor of a building.

Pollution levels can vary widely depending on where you live, ranging from urban cities to remote countryside. One way to find out the air pollution levels around your home is to check with your local authority or council and look at any air-quality status reports they may have published in the past year. Search for online resources such as apps you can download or websites that tell you your local air quality. These often allow you to view specific pollutants to check the level of emissions in your local area, and can be a great tool to use if you are particularly concerned about one specific type of pollutant. For example, you could check the nitrogen dioxide levels (given off from the combustion of fossil fuels from gas, coal or petrol

cars), which have been linked to many respiratory diseases.

If you live in a highly polluted area, such as near a busy road, consider using air filtration methods and only open your windows at night or outside of rush hours, when there is less traffic. If possible, you could also grow a hedge in front of your house; research has found that a beech hedge can reduce up to 50% of particulate matter, as well as cutting carbon monoxide and nitrogen dioxide.

If the air quality in your area is good, open your windows and create an airflow through your house at least once a day, even in winter. This will help flush out any stale air, balance moisture levels, and make you feel more alert and energized.

Your distance from the road or other contaminating sources can have a large impact on the air in your home.

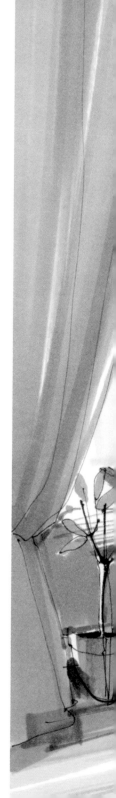

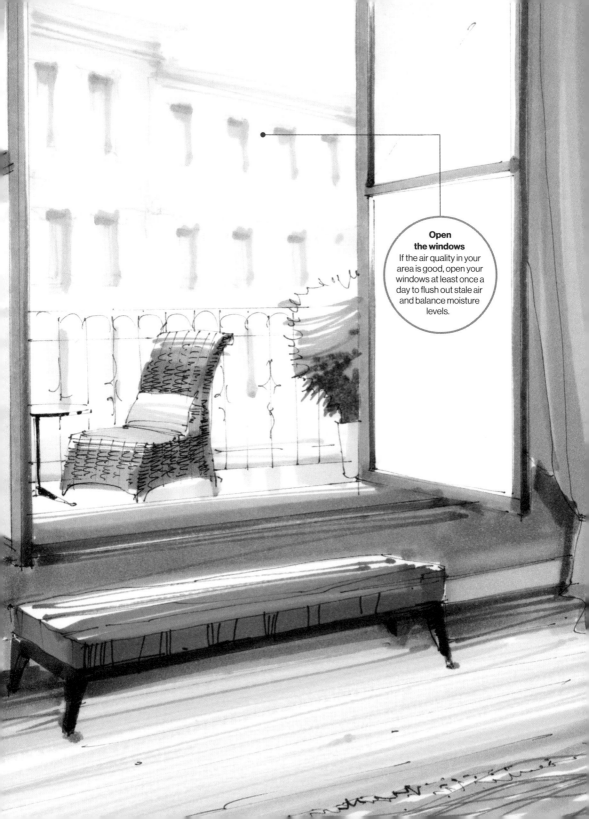

**Open
the windows**
If the air quality in your area is good, open your windows at least once a day to flush out stale air and balance moisture levels.

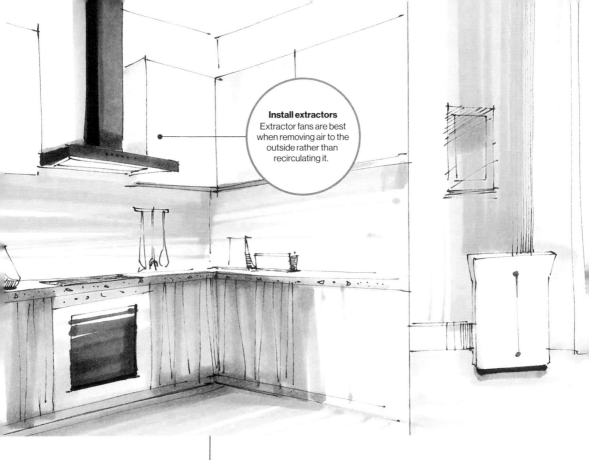

73 | Use air filtration

Access to clean air is vital for our health and wellbeing, and is essential for a healthy home. If you are concerned about indoor pollution, there are several air filtration methods you can try. These can help with bad odours, humidity and VOCs (volatile organic compounds), and help keep your lungs healthy.

Many older homes circulate fresh air through a system called natural ventilation, which relies on pressure differences in the building to draw airflow through small cracks, draughty windows or chimneys. Because many modern homes are air sealed for energy efficiency, this method isn't always possible, so we need to consider other ways to circulate airflow.

Mechanical ventilation systems can be used to pull stale air out and supply clean, fresh air back in by the use of ducts or fans. A typical example is an extractor fan unit, which works well in spaces that have higher humidity levels, such as bathrooms and kitchens.

Good ventilation systems can be costly, but they're a worthwhile investment; not only do

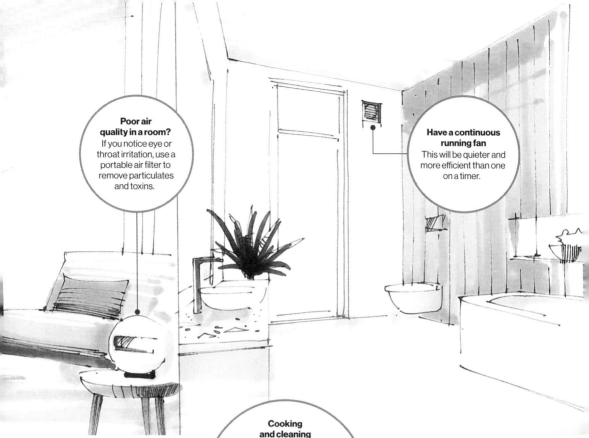

Poor air quality in a room?
If you notice eye or throat irritation, use a portable air filter to remove particulates and toxins.

Have a continuous running fan
This will be quieter and more efficient than one on a timer.

Cooking and cleaning
In one study, researchers opened windows after cooking and cleaning, then measured the indoor air quality after 15 and 30 minutes. Toxic particles had clung to walls and surfaces, rather than being diluted. This shows the need for mechanical ventilation.

they improve the air quality of the room, but they also save you money, since the long-term effects of high humidity levels can damage walls, ceilings and furniture.

If you live in an area with poor air quality, an air purifier should be a priority. These are available in different sizes, scales and costs.

Whole-home heat recovery systems – these systems extract stale, moist air from any room with water use, such as bathrooms and kitchens, then extract the warmth from it to preheat the fresh air being brought back in. The fresh air is run through filters before being pumped into all living spaces in the home. It can also be used to help cool a home during

warmer months. This type of system is costly and requires good duct runs, but is very effective.

Free-standing or floor-standing air filtering units can be plugged in and moved around the house to help filter the air by removing a variety of household odours, fumes, particulates and airborne toxins. Most do this using a high-efficiency particulate air (HEPA) filter. These smaller units are ideal for renters or for those who cannot undertake a major retrofit of their heating system. Look out for units designed with a quiet mode or low-noise features, which can be used in bedrooms to improve the air you breathe while you sleep.

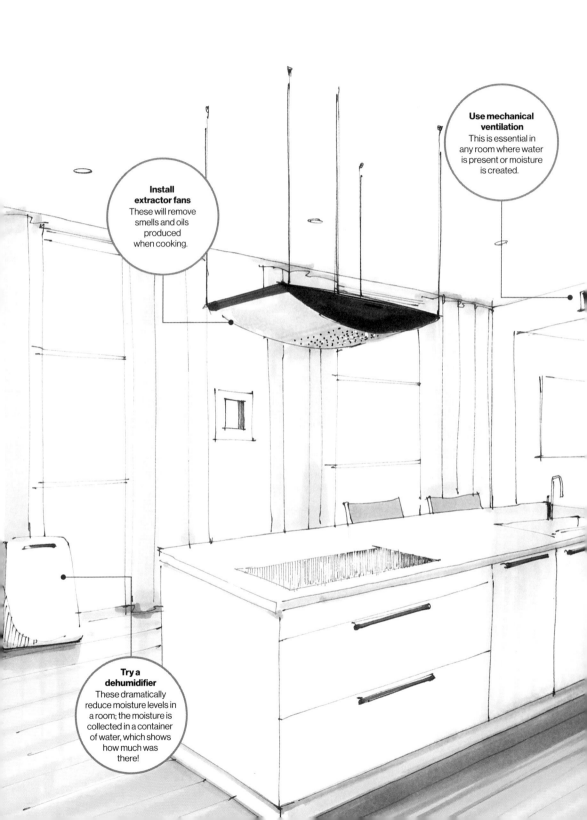

Install extractor fans
These will remove smells and oils produced when cooking.

Use mechanical ventilation
This is essential in any room where water is present or moisture is created.

Try a dehumidifier
These dramatically reduce moisture levels in a room; the moisture is collected in a container of water, which shows how much was there!

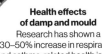

74 Prevent damp and mould

A build-up of mould in the home can not only look unappealing, but can also cause health problems – in fact, the World Health Organization calls it "microbial pollution".

But how can you prevent it? First, let's look at why it occurs and where to look out for it. Simply put, damp and mould are the result of excess moisture in the home. This can be caused by a number of factors: leaky roofs, broken water pipes, damaged window frames, blocked gutters, rising damp, fresh wet plaster drying out in a new-build home, or even damp clothes being left to dry on radiators.

Mould thrives in moist conditions and festers when there's a lack of ventilation, appropriate heating and insulation. This is why we tend to see a rise in outbreaks of mould in winter, when we close our windows to stay warm. Without this ventilation, the air turns stagnant and humid, encouraging condensation to build up inside and, in turn, mould forms.

As well as the ventilation solutions on pages 148–9, here are some things you could consider doing to help prevent microbial pollution such as damp and mould.

- **Open the windows** when you're having a shower or cooking hot, steamy dishes.
- **Retrofit an air vent** onto your windows.
- **Fix the source of the damp**, for example a blocked gutter or broken down pipe.
- **Invest in a dehumidifier** to dramatically lower moisture levels – you'll be amazed by how much moisture it draws out, even within an hour or so.
- **Dry your clothes outdoors** or use an energy-efficient tumble dryer.
- **Fix, replace or clean** your clogged-up kitchen extractor fan.
- **Fit continuous running extractor fans**, which can be very effective and energy efficient; remember to choose quieter models.

If mould has already started to grow, there are many natural ways to get rid of it without using toxic chemicals (see pages 156–7).

Health effects of damp and mould
Research has shown a 30–50% increase in respiratory and asthma-related health issues when damp and mould are present, and at least 20% of buildings in Europe, Canada and the United States has one or more signs of dampness.

75 | Remove dust and mites

Where do we start with dust? One day you wipe your shelves and chest of drawers, and the next day you see that thin, grey, fluffy layer has come right back. Dust appears for all kinds of reasons, and when it builds up, aside from making our spaces look a little unkempt, it can cause a lot of discomfort for many allergy sufferers.

Unwanted symptoms such as wheezing, eye irritation and itching can all be caused by dust mites – tiny organisms found in household dust – which are one of the biggest causes of allergic reactions. Luckily, there are many ways you can reduce the amount of dust in your home and continue to feel comfortable in your favourite spaces.

If you suffer from a dust-mite allergy, consider opting for hard flooring instead of carpets wherever possible. Dust mites tend to dwell and get trapped in textured carpets, and hard surfaces are easier to wipe down. If you already have carpets and you'd like to keep them, think about purchasing and regularly using a vacuum cleaner that is designed to trap more dust with high-efficiency particulate air (HEPA) filters.

Another way to keep on top of dust is to wash cushion covers, bed sheets, throws and pet bedding on a regular basis and at a high temperature to kill off any nasty bugs.

When cleaning surfaces, try using a damp cloth to help capture dust and discourage it from circulating in the air. Dust mites also thrive in humid environments, so try and keep the humidity below 50% (see page 151 for suggestions).

Lastly, consider fitting roller blinds instead of drapes or curtains, as they are easier to keep clean and wipe down, preventing dust mites from nestling into the fabric. Follow these tips and you'll be sure to notice a difference.

Use a damp cloth to help capture dust and discourage it from circulating in the air.

HOW TO KEEP DUST AT BAY

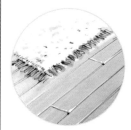

Hard flooring with a rug is easier to clean than wall-to-wall carpet.

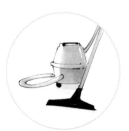

Choose a vacuum cleaner with high-efficiency particulate air (HEPA) filters to trap dust.

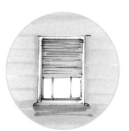

Roller blinds are easier to wipe down and clean to stop dust mites moving in.

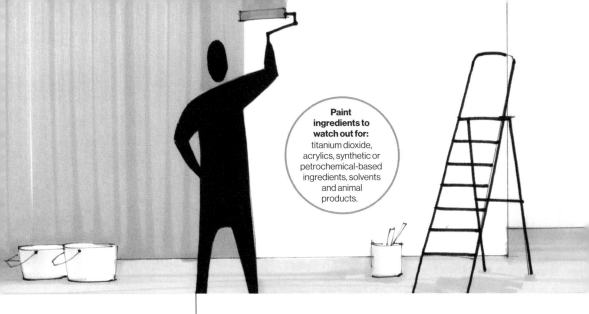

Paint ingredients to watch out for: titanium dioxide, acrylics, synthetic or petrochemical-based ingredients, solvents and animal products.

76 | Choose natural or eco paints

Painting your home is one of the most likely causes of air-quality problems in your home, either when you move in or after a refresh, so it's good to know what the healthier options are.

When you buy paint, a voluntary labelling system is in place to help you understand its contents.

Conventional (and often cheaper) paints are made with petrochemicals to improve their application and durability, but this comes at a cost. These paints often contain chemicals that will release gas as they dry, sending the toxic particulates into the air.

Although emulsion paints generally have fewer VOCs (volatile organic compounds), the oil-based gloss or eggshell versions can cause problems. If you move into a home that has a strong freshly painted room smell, it will be releasing VOCs. To get rid of this, ventilate the space well, open windows and use trays of activated charcoal or baking soda dotted around the room to soak up the smell overnight.

Luckily, there are a growing number of eco paints available that supply ultra-low or nontoxic versions. These are perfect for reducing toxins in the home, especially useful in rooms with typically less ventilation, for example the bedroom. Look out for labels such as the zero VOC label, the European Eco label or the Nordic Eco label.

Other good options might include:
• **clay paints**, which are breathable and let moisture in and out of walls – great for older properties.
• **casein paint** made from milk proteins and white lime; again good for older properties.
• **mineral-based paints** that contain pure potassium silicate or sodium silicate, which are highly durable and often applied to historic buildings.

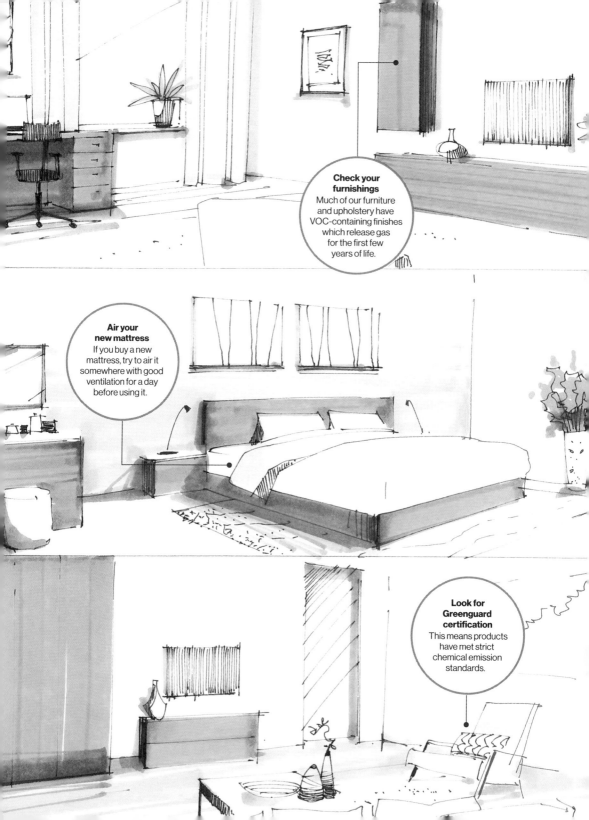

Check your furnishings
Much of our furniture and upholstery have VOC-containing finishes which release gas for the first few years of life.

Air your new mattress
If you buy a new mattress, try to air it somewhere with good ventilation for a day before using it.

Look for Greenguard certification
This means products have met strict chemical emission standards.

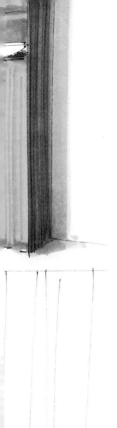

77 | Go for toxin-free furniture

Many porous household items, such as furniture and upholstery, absorb VOCs (volatile organic compounds) or have potentially toxic finishes applied to them during the manufacturing process, such as fire retardants. For the first few years of their life, these release gas (also called "off-gassing"), much like paint, and can be a catalyst for allergic reactions, causing irritation and even serious health problems after continued exposure.

Likely sources of toxic furniture and fittings in our homes include armchairs, mattresses, couches, carpets and any furniture made from MDF. Some of the most widely used toxins include formaldehyde (found in paints and adhesives), fire retardants, benzene (used in furniture manufacture), toluene (in foam mattresses) and phenylcyclohexane (in carpets). You can sometimes identify them by that distinctive "new-product" smell when you open the packaging. However, they can also be odourless and difficult to detect, which is why VOCs can be 2–5 times higher indoors than out.

Thankfully, there are several ways to reduce your exposure to indoor toxins and thus improve the air quality in your home. First, increase the ventilation in your house to help remove any VOCs (see page 148–9). When purchasing new products, consider choosing no- or low-VOC items or look for a Greenguard certification, which ensures they meet strict chemical emission standards. Alternatively, you can vacuum products regularly to draw out and remove toxins.

If none of these options are possible, try to ventilate the item when it arrives at your home by taking it out of its packaging and leaving it outside under shelter or in a well-ventilated room for at least 24 hours.

Consider second-hand products

These will have released most of their toxins already. You can find great-quality and unique pre-loved, antique, vintage or retro furniture – but do ensure they have the relevant fire safety labels.

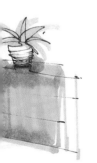

78 | Use non-toxic cleaning products

Even with busy lives and hectic schedules, cleaning our home is still a top priority. Not only does cleaning keep it looking tidy on the surface, but it also removes dust and allergens, which in turn promotes many health benefits. Unfortunately, many common household cleaning products contain harmful toxins that can contribute to serious health issues over prolonged usage.

In order to maintain a healthy, safe haven for you and your family, here are some products to look out for, and some to avoid. First, although the smell of bleach is associated with a clean home, it can be highly dangerous, especially if mixed with other chemicals such as ammonia. Bleach contains chlorine, which is corrosive to the lungs, skin and eyes, and can cause headaches, blurred vision, nausea and muscle weakness. For stubborn stains, try

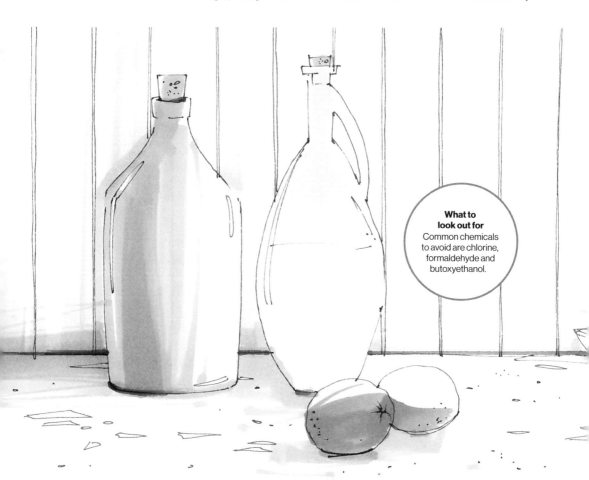

What to look out for
Common chemicals to avoid are chlorine, formaldehyde and butoxyethanol.

using baking soda and white vinegar (this also acts as a natural whitener if added to washes).

Other common chemicals to avoid are formaldehyde, found in heavy-duty cleaning products and a known carcinogen and VOC (volatile organic compound), and butoxyethanol, recognizable by its sweet scent in multi-purpose cleaners. Both of these can be harmful to the human body.

Instead, choose natural cleaning products, as they are much less polluting and contain fewer irritants. There are really effective natural cleaning products on the market, some of which can make you feel as though you're having aromatherapy while you use them.

You could even make your own cleaning products. Most things around the home can

Choose natural cleaning products, as they are much less polluting and contain fewer irritants.

be cleaned using a combination of white vinegar, baking soda, grape seed oil, eucalyptus oil, essential oils and citrus fruit, such as orange oil and lemon juice. Create your own combinations and preferred scents, then bottle them up in reusable spray bottles so they're always on hand. You could also check out castile soap, which is so non-toxic you can use it on your body!

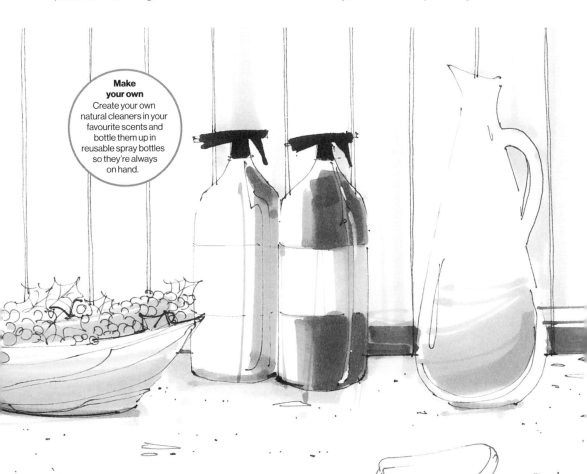

Make your own
Create your own natural cleaners in your favourite scents and bottle them up in reusable spray bottles so they're always on hand.

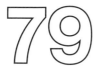

Use natural scents

Most of us have an incredibly refined sense of smell. Scents are highly personal, so when scenting our homes it's really important to consider everyone living there, as preferences and tolerance levels can vary hugely.

In the home, we might be using sprays, atomizers and scented candles to bring different aromas into our spaces. However, these methods of indoor scenting can introduce additional VOCs (volatile organic compounds) into the air in the home, and unfortunately, although we all love the atmosphere created by a flickering candle, they release ultra-fine particulate matter (PM 2.5) into the air.

Some scenting products are more harmful than others. Phthalates, which have been linked to problems with reproduction, can be found lurking in many fragranced household products, such as air fresheners. You won't always see phthalates listed on the label, since by law companies don't have to disclose their scents. However, the word "fragrance" in the ingredients list often indicates that phthalates are there.

HOME SCENTING IDEAS

If you're keen to introduce scents into your home, try opting for natural scenting to keep the air as healthy as possible. Consider how you want to feel in each space and choose the scent accordingly; for example citrus to enliven, lavender to relax. Here are some suggestions.

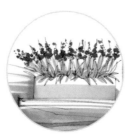

Use or make your own all-natural organic room sprays or misters.

Make your own potpourri (a mixture of dried, naturally fragrant plant materials).

Simmer spices with citrus fruit in a pan to create a warm aroma.

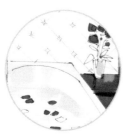

Grow scented plants inside, such as jasmine, gardenia, scented geraniums or pelargoniums, citrus plants, tea rose begonias, lavender, fragrant orchids, pansy orchids, *Stephanotis floribunda* (Madagascar jasmine) or paperwhite narcissi.

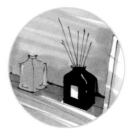

Float scented leaves in a bowl of water to create a natural air freshener, as well as visual interest.

Display cut herbs and flowers – either in water, or by hanging them to dry out.

Use an ultrasonic aromatherapy diffuser: add water and essential oil, then enjoy the gentle wafts of mist.

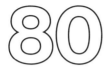

Manage seasonal allergies

With seasonal allergies on the increase due to a rise in air-quality problems, increased carbon dioxide levels and warmer temperatures, more of us are suffering. Many of the suggestions throughout this section will help reduce the triggers for allergic conditions, as will reducing stress and getting restful sleep, but there are extra things you can do to alleviate allergy symptoms.

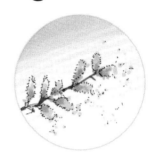

Being aware of what triggers your allergy is the first step in creating a healthier home where reactions are kept to a minimum, so start by keeping an allergy diary to work out when they are triggered.

You may identify that at certain times of the year your symptoms are worse, and this will give you an insight into whether pollen or moulds trigger your body's reactions; for example:

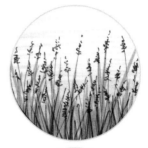

March to June: tree pollen
June to August/September: grass pollen
August to October: weed pollen
Autumn: outdoor moulds

The pollen count is highest between 5 and 10am and at dusk, so if you know which pollen triggers your allergic reaction, try to avoid exercising outside, opening windows or hanging out your washing at these times during the months when that pollen count is highest. Knowing what causes your reactions will also mean you can enjoy fresh air and being out in nature when the triggers are at their lowest.

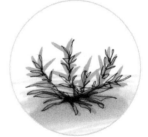

Indoor and outdoor air pollution can trigger allergy-induced asthma, and 10–30% of the global population suffer from allergic rhinitis.

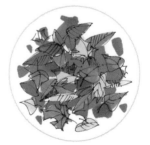

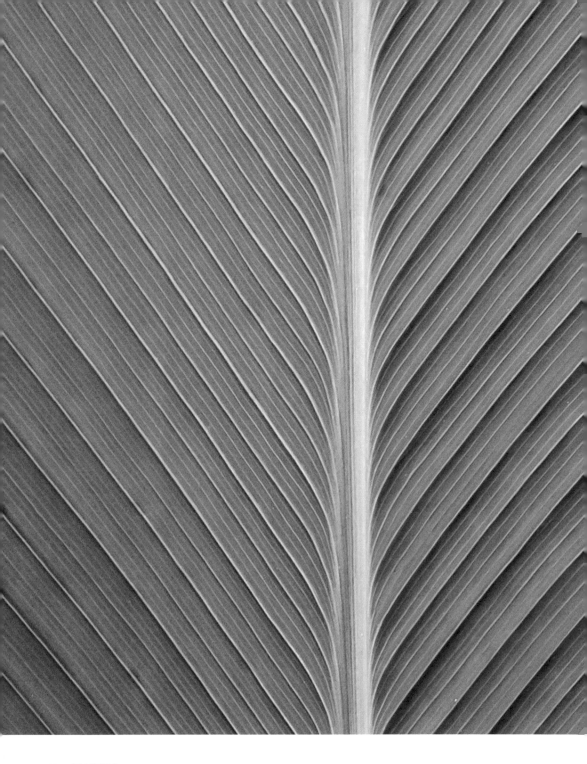

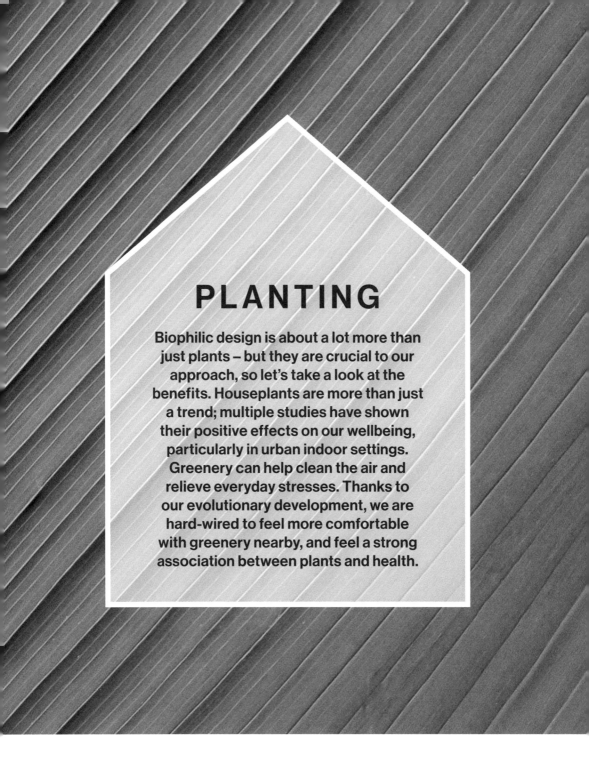

PLANTING

Biophilic design is about a lot more than just plants – but they are crucial to our approach, so let's take a look at the benefits. Houseplants are more than just a trend; multiple studies have shown their positive effects on our wellbeing, particularly in urban indoor settings. Greenery can help clean the air and relieve everyday stresses. Thanks to our evolutionary development, we are hard-wired to feel more comfortable with greenery nearby, and feel a strong association between plants and health.

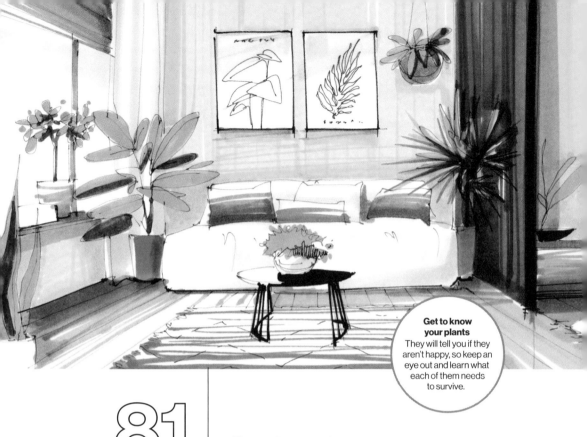

**Get to know
your plants**
They will tell you if they
aren't happy, so keep an
eye out and learn what
each of them needs
to survive.

81 | Caring for plants

Many people are worried that houseplants might be tricky to care for.
But they can boost our vitality, productivity and creativity – surely it's
worth learning how to care for them, so they can nurture you back?

Here are some top tips to ensure your plants look lush all year round, stay alive and grow alongside you. Don't be surprised if you become quite attached to your favourite plants as you help them thrive over a lifetime!

The first thing to remember is that most houseplants are from tropical regions, so are accustomed to shady jungle floors, under thick, leafy canopies. This is not so different from our warm houses shaded by rooftops, so these plants are quite happy to live indoors with us. But if you're not green fingered and feel intimidated, start slowly and consider investing in low-maintenance plants such as cacti or succulents.

If you struggle to remember to water plants, consider working it into your routine by creating a fixed time each week when you do the watering rounds. Setting a reminder on your phone will help you forge a habit. You could even create a watering schedule and nominate a different person each week; this can be a nice way to get everyone involved with plant care. Alternatively, you could think about investing in a self-watering device, if you're finding it hard to commit.

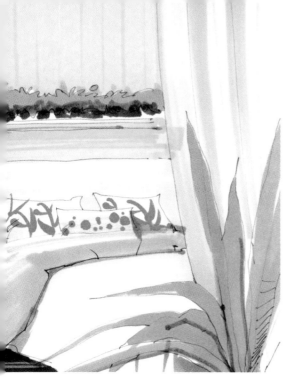

let it dry. You can also get very affordable soil moisture testers to help you know whether you are getting the moisture levels right. Alternatively, stick the tip of your finger into the soil about 2cm deep – if it feels dry, give it a drink, and if there is still some moisture, come back another day. To help your plants flourish, cut off any dead leaves so the plant's energy is not wasted on them. This also speeds up growth spurts.

Plants are good at letting us know if they aren't happy. Too much or too little of anything, and they'll start to look a little sad, so keep an eye out for signs of distress. If your plant isn't getting enough light, the leaves may turn yellow or drop off, leaf growth may be stunted (fewer new leaves and smaller ones when they do grow), or stems might grow longer as they try to reach for the light. Variegated leaves (those with more than one colour) can turn plain green, or bright green leaves can dull or turn brown. Try moving it to a sunnier spot in the room, or to a south-facing room. If it has too much direct sun or not enough water, leaves can dry out and turn brown. It's a balancing act! If you're not sure, look up its preferences and where it originates from, and hopefully it will become clear.

Although plants need water to survive, they can have too much. If a plant's roots stay damp for too long, they can rot and the leaves may turn yellow. Make sure it isn't drowning – if your plant is in a pot with drainage holes, but inside another vessel or dish, chances are it could be sitting in a puddle, so tip that out and

PLANT CARE TIPS

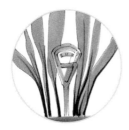

Use a water meter – just stick this in the soil and instantly get a moisture level reading.

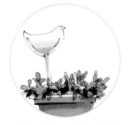

A watering device will slowly release moisture into the soil – perfect if you've been known to forget about plant watering.

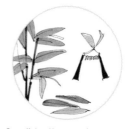

Cut off dead leaves – these waste your plant's energy, so remove them to help it thrive.

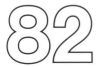

82 | Analyse your light levels

The light conditions in your home play a big role in the upkeep of your plants. As a plant receives light, water and carbon dioxide it photosynthesizes (in other words, converts the light energy into food) and then, in turn, it grows.

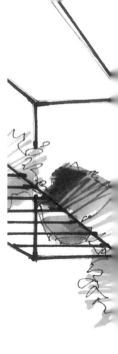

Plants have varying optimal lighting conditions: some cannot survive in direct sunlight, while others flourish there. Cacti like direct sunlight and can tolerate very little water because their native habitat is desert with very little shade. On the other hand, the leaves of cast-iron plants, traditionally found low on the forest floors of Japan, will scorch in direct sunlight.

When positioning your plant in a room, the distance from the main light source can have a large impact. Even if you think a room has a lot of light, you still need to consider exactly where you put a plant, depending on its needs – to a plant, the shadiest corner of a room is totally different to the windowsill. Either might work for the right plant.

The human eye automatically adjusts when receiving light, which makes it difficult for us to identify subtle differences in light levels. In order to quantify the light intensity accurately, consider investing in a light meter that measures in either foot candles or lux, or download a plant-orientated light meter app for your smart phone. Then, pick the spot where you'd like your plant to live and measure the lighting conditions throughout the day, taking note of how many hours of light it would receive there in comparison to other locations. Most houseplants will tolerate light levels ten times lower than their ideal range, but probably won't thrive. Without this technology, it may be more a matter of trial and error, selecting a spot you think would be suitable and trying your plant out there. It will soon tell you if it's not happy!

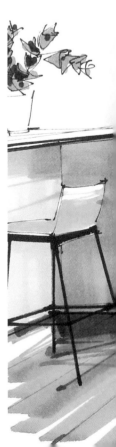

How much light do plants need?
As a loose guideline, low-light plants need 500–2,500 lux, medium-light plants 2,500–10,000 lux, bright light plants 10,000–20,000 lux, and very bright-light plants need about 20,000–50,000 lux.

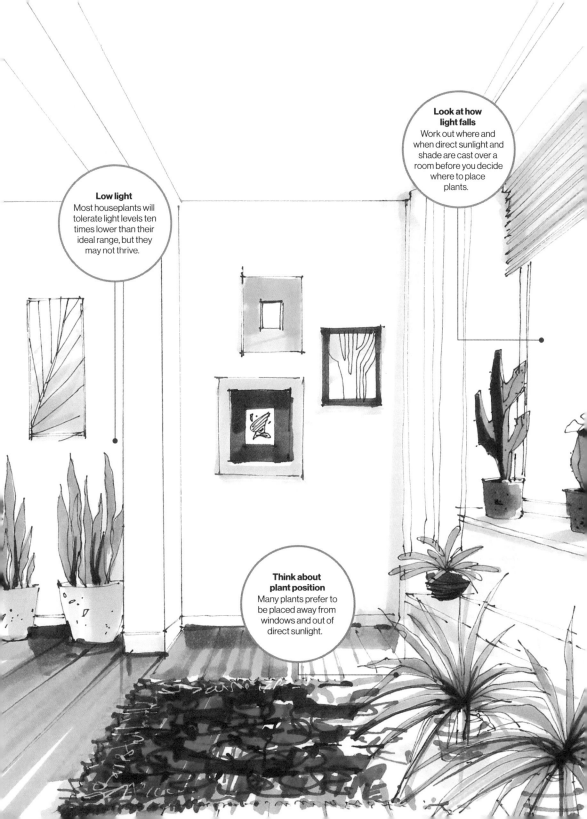

Look at how light falls
Work out where and when direct sunlight and shade are cast over a room before you decide where to place plants.

Low light
Most houseplants will tolerate light levels ten times lower than their ideal range, but they may not thrive.

Think about plant position
Many plants prefer to be placed away from windows and out of direct sunlight.

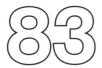

Introduce tabletop plants

Positioning plants so that they're the centrepiece of your table is a great way to save floor space and create a focal point in your home, or to soften harder corners of a room. Their welcoming, lush appearance will draw people in around a dining table, and can brighten up any coffee table or sideboard. The presence of plants on tabletops brings them into your eye line, helping you to connect with natural systems like growth and the changing of the seasons.

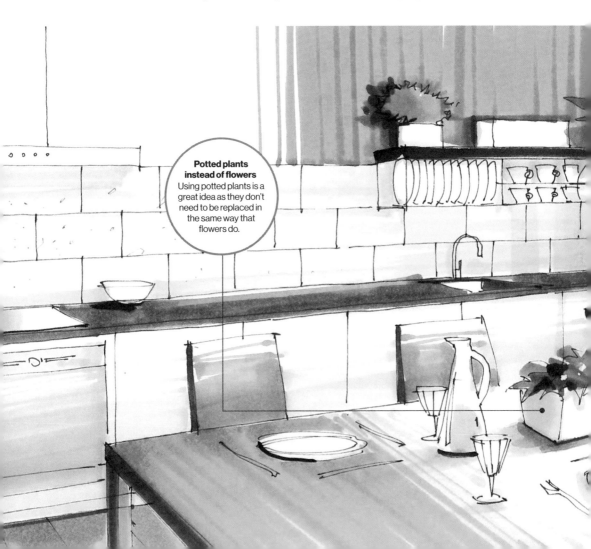

Potted plants instead of flowers
Using potted plants is a great idea as they don't need to be replaced in the same way that flowers do.

Consider choosing plants like *Oxalis triangularis* (false shamrock), which opens and closes in response to the amount of daylight, as this will connect you to the passing of time thanks to your plants' circadian rhythms!

Tabletop plants can also add texture, colour and pattern through your choice of pot, planter or container. If you prefer earthy, organic colour palettes, consider using natural, stripped-back materials like plain ceramic, clay or stone pots. If you love bold, primary tones, there's an opportunity here to include some pops of colour. If your home is traditional and you're an admirer of the Arts and Crafts movement, consider investing in a highly decorative pot. You could even commission a local ceramicist to make you something to pass on to the next generation.

The size of your plant is important too; consider if it will block views, eye contact between people or valuable light. You can also use tabletop plants to divide your space and create some visual and acoustic privacy.

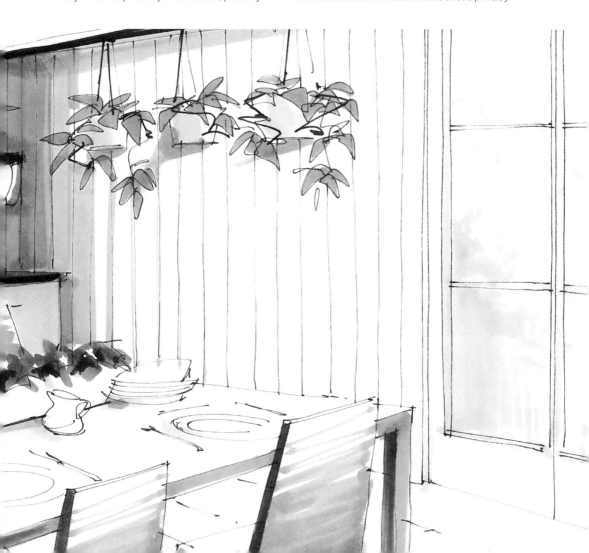

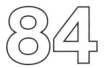

84 | Introduce floor plants

Pot plants positioned on the ground provide a great opportunity to create circulation routes and define zones within a room, while also softening hard edges and boundaries between spaces.

A good example of this is using a cluster of plants to create a screen or mini divide between two areas in a room. Using planting can be much cheaper and easier than fitting a structural, more permanent room divider like a screen, wall or shelving. What's more, it allows more flexibility and variation, as it can adapt as your needs or activities in the room change. One moment you may be working from home and need a small, private refuge for concentration, and the next you may want to move the plants to the perimeters of the space for a party.

Arranging plants with varying heights can create a more organic feel by imitating how plants would grow in a natural setting. You can achieve this by varying the size and type of plants in each cluster, as well as the pots, some of which you might raise on plant stands or small stools. Choosing natural materials such as weathered timber for your plinths will help boost your connection to nature.

When deciding which plants will occupy your floor, consider their leaf sizes and how they feel – your hands and legs may brush past floor plants more than other types. Soft, leafy or grassy and tactile plants would work well. Just make sure these easily reachable plants aren't toxic for children or pets who might get their hands or paws on them.

> **Using planting can be much cheaper and easier than fitting a structural, more permanent room divider.**

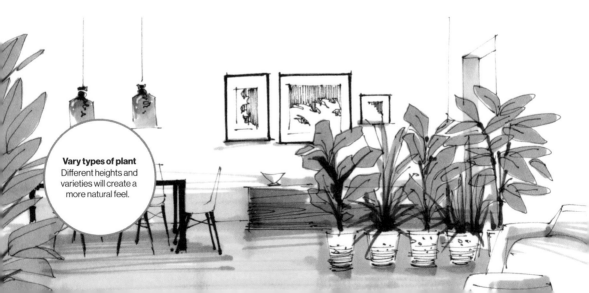

Vary types of plant
Different heights and varieties will create a more natural feel.

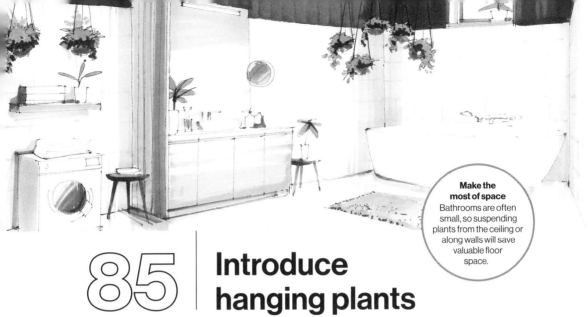

85 | Introduce hanging plants

Trailing and hanging plants are a great way to brighten up a room and breathe new life into your home. Growing vertically creates an amazing cascading effect, emphasizing tropical lushness and obscuring sightlines, which can create the sense of mystery you find in natural landscapes, cultivating curiosity and a desire to explore. High planting in your home recreates what we would experience in a jungle or forest habitat. To immerse yourself in a space full of life and greenery, put some of your plants up high.

Trailing plants not only look great, but are practical too. They help save valuable floor space between your furniture, if you are limited in this department. Positioning them either on high shelves or in hanging planters will also encourage the eye to gaze upwards and, as a result, make a space feel bigger. Just make sure that you can get easy, regular access in order to water and maintain the plant.

Consider using macramé plant hangers to suspend potted plants. These are easy to hang from rails or hooks and are a great way to bring additional textures and decoration into your home. If you are feeling crafty, look into making a *kokedama* (Japanese for moss ball). This is a root ball of earth that holds a plant, which is then wrapped in a layer of moss and bound together with string (or ideally waterproof fishing twine). These are enormously satisfying to make, have a natural, organic quality to them and look great suspended in a cluster. Instructions for making both macramé plant hangers and *kokedama* are available online.

Bringing high planting into your home recreates what we would experience in a jungle or forest habitat.

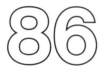

86 | Create a mini green wall

Green walls are a great way to introduce plants to your home and are now becoming more affordable. Like hanging plants, they look lush and welcoming and save on floor space. They are also great for absorbing noise, making them ideal for apartment living, or if you have noisy neighbours.

Thanks to the density of greenery in a green wall, they are one of the best ways to improve air quality through the plants' ability to absorb carbon dioxide and toxins in the home, such as VOCs (volatile organic compounds), benzene and formaldehyde, depending on which plants you include.

Although commercial green wall systems require water supplies and drainage, you can now buy self-contained systems for domestic use. These systems are no-fuss and easy to use: you simply install it onto your wall, add your chosen plants, then make sure you top up the integral water reservoir system every so often. When choosing a position for your green wall, don't forget to consider the natural light levels and which plants will work best here, too.

An alternative system is a felt-pocket planting system for green walls. You can easily move and replace plants, which is good if you like to experiment with different looks or colour schemes. However, as there is no reservoir system of water, moisture is controlled by the soil and felt's ability to retain it, so more careful maintenance may be required.

Green walls are great for absorbing noise, making them ideal for apartment living or if you have noisy neighbours.

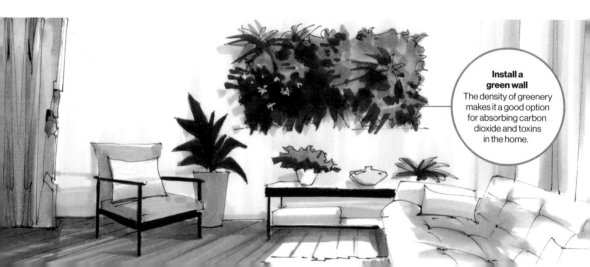

Install a green wall
The density of greenery makes it a good option for absorbing carbon dioxide and toxins in the home.

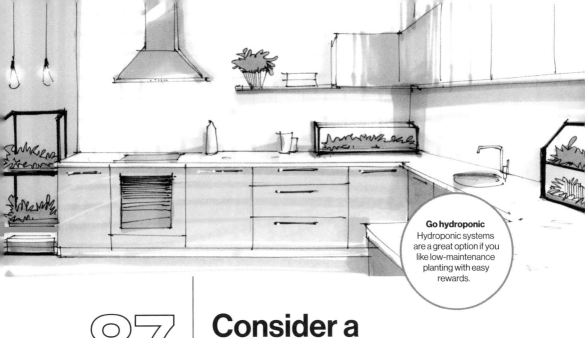

Go hydroponic
Hydroponic systems are a great option if you like low-maintenance planting with easy rewards.

87 | Consider a hydroponic system

A hydroponic system is an innovative technological solution for growing plants in artificial light and without the use of soil. As we know, plants need nutrients and water to grow, and most of them get this from soil. In a hydroponic system, the nutrients are instead dissolved into the water to be absorbed. The plants are either misted, flooded or suspended in the nutrient-rich water, which is pH-balanced perfectly to suit their needs. They generally use an integrated artificial lighting system, so there's no need to worry about having enough natural light.

Hydroponic systems for use in the home are becoming more widely available, as more people want to grow their own vegetables with limited or non-existent garden space. This growing trend is not only mess free, but also allows you to grow all year round. On top of this, it's a great option if you like low-maintenance planting with easy rewards. Hydroponic systems create optimal growing conditions for your plants to thrive in, so it's easy to produce quick results.

You can grow almost anything using a hydroponic system – the only difference is the method by which the plants receive nutrients and their method of stability. Smaller plants such as basil don't need a big support system, so they are sometimes grown in a glass jar. Larger plants that normally anchor themselves deeply in soil, such as spider plants or devil's ivy, may need the help of pumice stones or stone wool plugs to keep them growing upright towards the light.

If you're a beginner, you can choose a kit that does a lot of the legwork for you. With some kits, you will need to manually control the settings, while some will automatically water your plants and work out the light based on a timer, so you really can plug in and go.

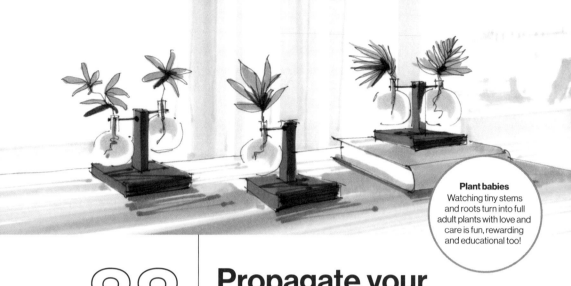

Plant babies
Watching tiny stems and roots turn into full adult plants with love and care is fun, rewarding and educational too!

Propagate your houseplants

Propagating houseplants is a great way cut down on plant miles and avoid the use of peat-based compost (intensive mining of peat bogs destroys the habitat of plants, insects and birds that rely upon them). It's sustainable and costs nothing if you pot them in re-used containers, such as clean food tins, using homemade compost. You can give cuttings away as homegrown gifts, or swap them for other plants with people in your community.

Not all houseplants are suitable for propagating but, luckily, many varieties are. Do a bit of background research to find out if your plant is suitable and what propagating method will best set you up for success.

A simple, effective method is to propagate your plants in water. Identify whether your chosen plant "mother" has root nodes (the bumpy areas on the stem). If yours does, make a clean cut to take a section of stem

> **Do a bit of background research to find out which propagating method will best set you up for success.**

that includes a node. Try to cut this from an area of new growth, where you see a new baby leaf coming through. Pop it in a glass of water or clear container, then be patient until it starts to sprout roots. Change the water weekly and leave it in a bright spot, such as on your windowsill, but out of direct sunlight. Once the roots are about 1.5cm long (usually 3–4 weeks), they are ready to pot.

To pot your new plant, place some pre-moistened potting soil in the bottom of a small pot so that the roots are raised an inch or so from the base. Once your plant is resting in there, fill in the gaps around it with more moist soil. Water it well until the water runs out the bottom; drainage holes make this easier. Finally, place your new plant in a spot that will suit it, depending on its species.

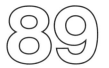

Try preserved plants

Although it's best to have real living elements of nature in your home, an alternative is to use preserved planting. It's not as dynamic as real plants, but it helps add natural patterns and texture, and is hassle free and long lasting.

Preserved planting, such as leaves, flowers, fronds and grasses, is now available in a wide variety of shapes and sizes. The plants have undergone a process which replaces the natural plant sap with a solution to preserve its freshness, scent and form for many years without the need for any maintenance, other than the occasional dusting.

You might also consider decorating your home with dried-out branches found on a woodland walk. Eucalyptus and willow branches are particularly captivating and look striking when displayed in a vase or wicker basket. Dried reeds and grasses found near a local pond will also bring natural textures and create a statement display.

Flowers look beautiful in full bloom, but preserved flowers have their own unique qualities and benefits. They save you money and help build a sense of familiarity and sentiment, as they last a long time. Using a simple book-pressing technique to dry out your flowers is the best-known method, or try hanging a bunch upside down.

Last on our list – for good reason – is artificial or plastic plants, sometimes called faux plants. They can look incredibly realistic and are available in an ever-growing range, but remember that anyone who touches a fake plant may feel cheated by its artificiality, so they can have a negative effect. A good way to avoid this is to only use artificial plants in inaccessible areas, such as beyond barriers or high up in a space, and to combine them with real plants in areas where people may come into direct contact with them.

TYPES OF PRESERVED PLANT

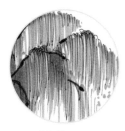

Dried leaves create an incredibly low-maintenance but natural statement display.

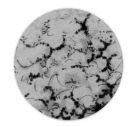

Preserved moss is a good way to add natural textures, patterns and colours; it's a halfway house between real and artificial plants.

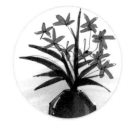

Artificial plants and flowers are now enormously convincing and are a good option where maintenance is difficult, such as high shelving.

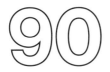

Take a room-by-room approach

Once you've decided to fill your home with plants, where should you start? Over the next few pages we have suggested varying styles and functions of plants for different rooms in the home. Combine these with our tips on analysing lighting levels (see page 164) to get the right mix of plants.

To start with, are your plants going to be functional or decorative? There are a number of plants that can enhance activities of specific rooms, such as relaxation, sleep or cooking. On the other hand, you might just want to add colour, texture, pattern or movement to a space.

Once you've decided this, where do you want to put them? If they are functional, you'll need to make sure there is space for these in the right places, such as a windowsill designated for a herb box. From a decorative perspective, you might want clusters of floor-standing plants, trailing plants on shelves, hanging plants or tabletop plants. If you have space, why not consider all of these options? You may even be tempted to make a statement with a green wall. Assess

If you plan where you want your plants to go, it will make it easier to choose which plants you can bring in.

the space you have on a room-by-room basis; if you plan where you want your plants to go, it will make it easier to choose which plants you can bring in.

In fact, why not picture your home right now and think of some spots in need of greenery? This should help you to create an idea of what you'd go for when reading through the suggestions that follow.

BEDROOM *see page 176 for more*

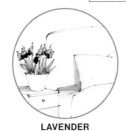

LAVENDER

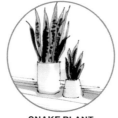

SNAKE PLANT

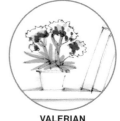

VALERIAN

KITCHEN & DINING ROOM *see page 179*

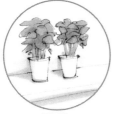

BASIL

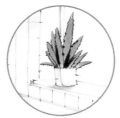

ALOE VERA

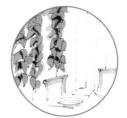

HEARTLEAF
PHILODENDRON

BATHROOM *see page 180*

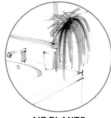

AIR PLANTS

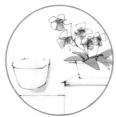

ORCHIDS

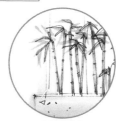

BAMBOO

LIVING ROOM *see page 183*

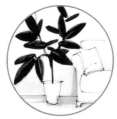

RUBBER TREE

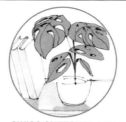

SWISS CHEESE PLANT

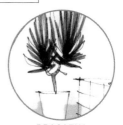

DRACAENA

HOME OFFICE *see page 184*

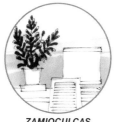

*ZAMIOCULCAS
ZAMIIFOLIA* (ZZ PLANT)

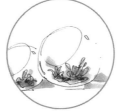

TERRARIUM

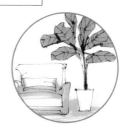

FIDDLE-LEAF FIG

91 | Add plants to bedrooms

Getting a good night's sleep is vital; it makes us feel restored, increases our productivity during the day and boosts our physical health and mental wellbeing. There are many common household plants that thrive indoors and have sleep-inducing qualities that can help us doze off. Here are a few, with their unique characteristics.

Lavender is best known for its therapeutic qualities and helping us rest; its aroma is commonly used as an essential oil for relaxation and aromatherapy. Not only does lavender bring a touch of colour to your room, but studies also tell us that smelling lavender before bed will help you fall into a deeper night's sleep, making you feel more energized the next morning.

Jasmine also releases a calming scent that is often used in aromatherapy. In fact, one study proved that its sweet, distinctive smell was as effective as some sedatives and sleeping pills. Be sure to water your jasmine plant frequently during its flowering periods, and less so in non-flowering periods.

Valerian not only looks beautiful, but if you struggle to unwind and drift off, its scent can induce sleep when inhaled. While valerian is traditionally used an as oral sleep aid, you could consider sprinkling some petals into your evening bath too.

Aloe vera, like many houseplants, can improve our sleep quality by releasing oxygen at night and absorbing the carbon dioxide we breathe out, making it well suited for bedrooms. It loves being placed on a bright windowsill, as it thrives in direct sunlight.

Peace lilies, like their name suggests, work hard to care for us. Not only are they blessed with beautiful white flowers in full bloom, but they also have powerful air cleaning characteristics and, similarly to aloe vera, release oxygen at night while we sleep. Peace lilies can increase the humidity levels of your bedroom by up to 5%, which may help you avoid dry skin and colds.

Snake plants, also known as mother-in-law's tongue, are another front-runner for your bedroom plant collection. They are super hardy and very hard to kill off. Because they tolerate low light conditions, they are ideal for homes that lack natural light. What makes them good for bedrooms in particular is that they release oxygen at night, helping us fall into a deep slumber and wake up feeling refreshed.

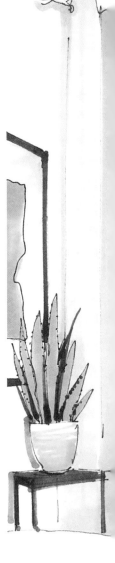

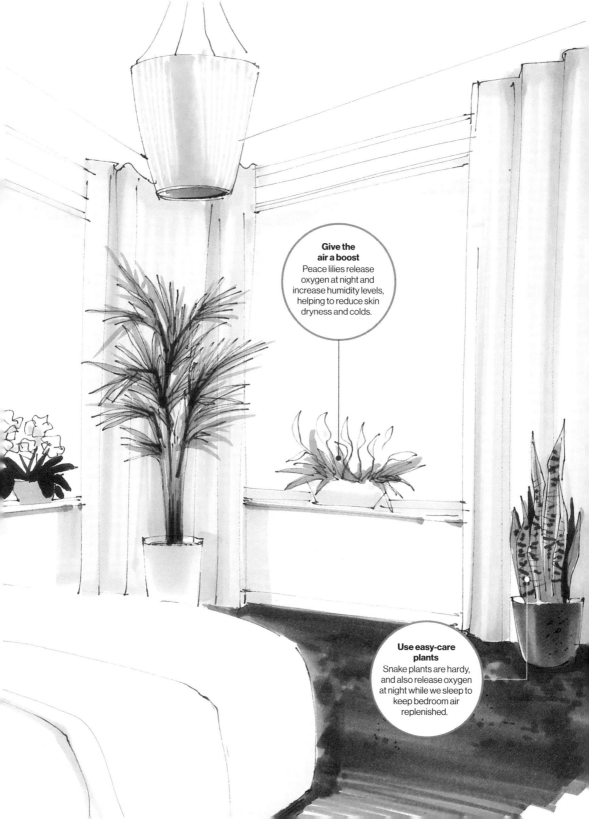

Give the air a boost
Peace lilies release oxygen at night and increase humidity levels, helping to reduce skin dryness and colds.

Use easy-care plants
Snake plants are hardy, and also release oxygen at night while we sleep to keep bedroom air replenished.

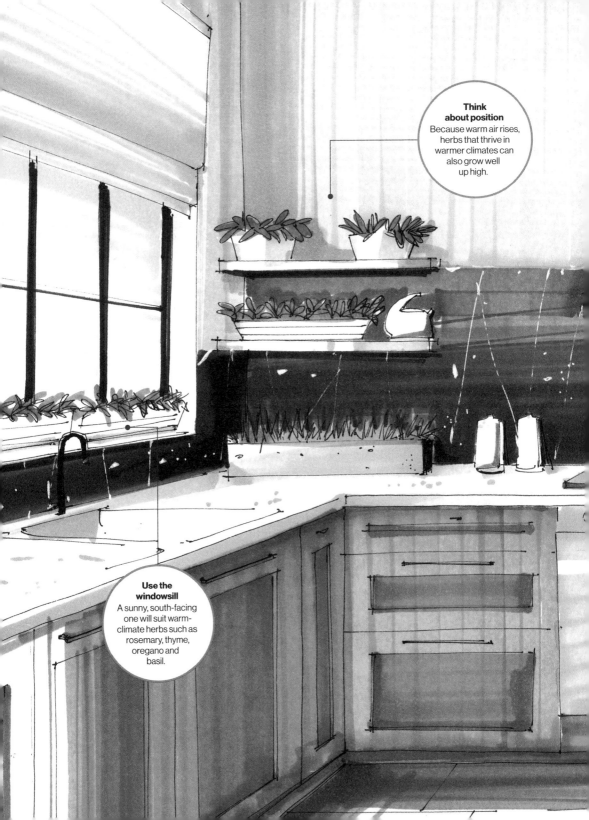

Think about position
Because warm air rises, herbs that thrive in warmer climates can also grow well up high.

Use the windowsill
A sunny, south-facing one will suit warm-climate herbs such as rosemary, thyme, oregano and basil.

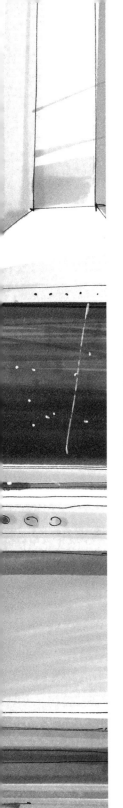

92 | Add plants to the kitchen

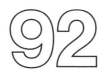

If you are limited on garden space and love having herbs easily accessible for cooking, growing herbs in your kitchen is probably for you. Growing edible plants inside has lots of benefits; it not only saves you money and helps you make delicious, nutritious meals, but also adds visual richness and texture to your kitchen.

There is a huge variety of herbs, and many are happy to live on your countertop. Space can be in short supply, so use your windowsills.

Ideally, choose a shady, east-facing windowsill for herbs that prefer a cooler climate, such as **parsley**, **mint** and **chives**.

A sunny, south-facing windowsill is best for herbs that come from warm climates, such as **rosemary**, **thyme**, **oregano** and **basil**. When positioning these sun lovers, check to see if any trees or roof overhangs cast shade.

If so, consider moving them to another, sunnier spot.

Because warm air rises, herbs that thrive in warmer climates can grow well up high. If your kitchen is in a basement and receives very little light, you could even consider purchasing a grow light. This clever piece of technology will create ideal light conditions for your herbs to thrive in.

Other good choices are **aloe vera**, which helps soothe burns, in the kitchen, and **heartleaf philodendron** for a dining room centrepiece.

Growing edible plants saves you money, helps you make delicious, nutritious meals, and adds visual richness and texture.

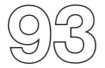

Add plants to the bathroom

With their proven record for reducing stress, plants are a great addition to your bathroom, and will help create a lush, green oasis to emphasize that sense of retreat. Along with easy access to water (handy for watering schedules), the bathroom, with its high humidity levels, offers the perfect conditions for many moisture-loving plants to thrive.

Snake plants' ability to tolerate low light make them a popular choice for the bathroom, as many of them are quite lacking in natural light. They also thrive in high humidity.

If you are limited on space in your bathroom, consider planting **pothos**, also known as money plant or devil's ivy, in hanging planters. Pothos can handle low light levels, thrives in humid environments and grows rapidly, so you'll have your bathroom jungle in no time.

You could also create a beautiful display of suspended **air plants** in decorative vessels overhead or along the walls – they are easy to look after and very hardy.

If you have generous floor space and want to create a zen-like atmosphere, think about growing **bamboo** in a container. Bamboo's height also makes it effective for screening off certain areas and creating subtle divides.

Cast-iron plants (also called aspidistra) are another household favourite, as they are very hard to kill and can tolerate most conditions. Cast-iron plants are low maintenance; they don't require a lot of watering, so wait for the soil to dry out before you tend to your plant again.

Alternatively, if you're looking for flowering plants that can survive in the bathroom, consider an **orchid**. Since they are native to tropical humid climates, they will thrive in the steamy conditions.

Aloe vera has amazing healing qualities, making it ideally situated in your bathroom, where it can provide a quick, soothing remedy for sunburn or insect bites.

Rotate your plants
If your bathroom has no window, remember that you can move plants around your home. They can come to visit for a few days before being moved back to a lighter, brighter space. If you continue this rotation and have enough plants, you'll always have a lush, green bathroom.

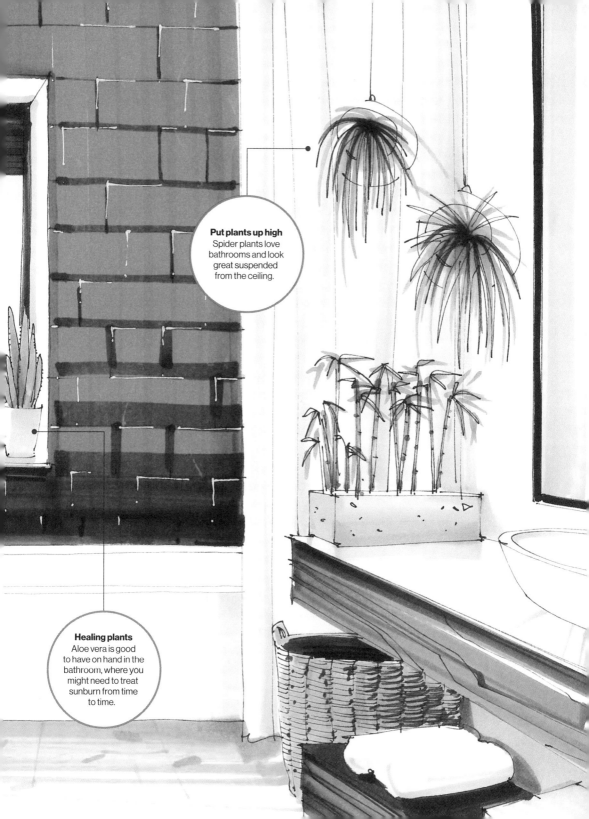

Put plants up high
Spider plants love bathrooms and look great suspended from the ceiling.

Healing plants
Aloe vera is good to have on hand in the bathroom, where you might need to treat sunburn from time to time.

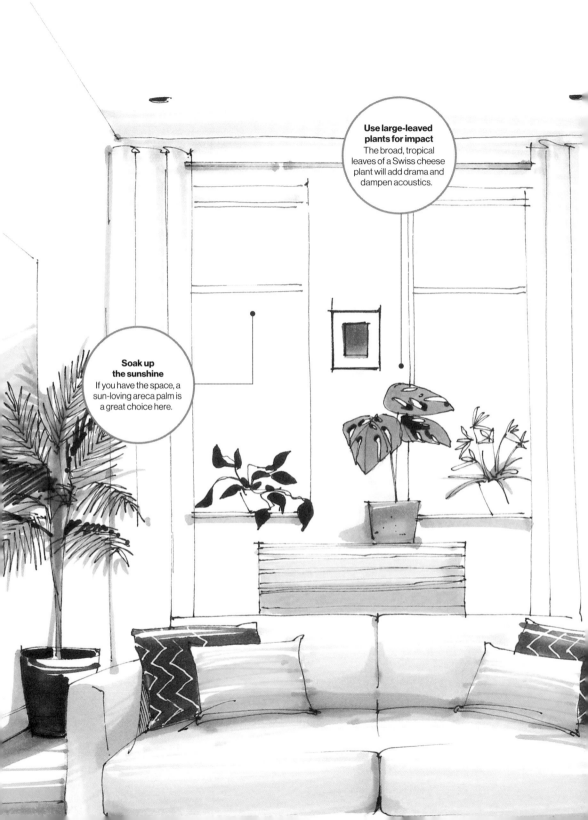

Use large-leaved plants for impact
The broad, tropical leaves of a Swiss cheese plant will add drama and dampen acoustics.

Soak up the sunshine
If you have the space, a sun-loving areca palm is a great choice here.

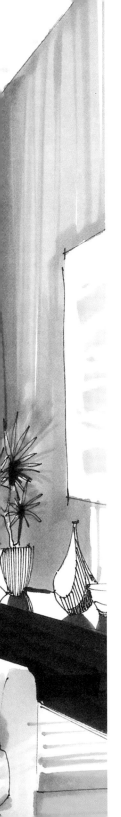

94 Add plants to the living room

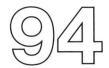

Surrounding yourself with plants in your living room adds life and pops of colour, as well as boosting your mood and creativity levels. Many plants also work hard to detoxify the air we breathe, removing indoor air pollutants and helping create a healthy living environment. In order to reap the benefits of this, you need quite a lot of plants, so consider a combination of these suggestions.

If you have a south-facing window providing bright sunlight, consider housing a **rubber plant**. These are known for their beautiful, leathery, deep maroon leaves and their amazing formaldehyde-removing qualities. They thrive in direct sunlight, but they're pretty tough and versatile, and will tolerate lower light conditions too.

If you are limited on natural light and space, **pothos** is a great choice again here. Aside from tolerating low light and being beautiful to hang overhead or from shelves, it sits at the top of the list for plants that remove indoor air toxins, as does the sun-loving **areca palm** (also known as a butterfly palm), which is a great choice if space isn't an issue.

Dracaenas can also cleanse the air, and are tall and lush, so they can add a little drama to your living room.

Finally, if you want to make a statement, then consider a ***Monstera deliciosa*** (also known as a cheese plant) or **bird of paradise**. Their broad, tropical leaves will liven up your home and help dampen acoustics.

Many plants work hard to detoxify the air we breathe, removing indoor air pollutants and helping create a healthy living space.

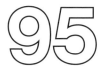

95 | Add plants to your workspace

If you work from home, staying stimulated, creative and motivated in your dedicated space is a priority. Indoor plants not only make your space more alive and engaging, but are also recognized for their productivity-boosting and stress-reducing abilities. Plants can produce cleaner air, which results in clearer thinking and helps prevent fatigue. Things tend to encroach on our desk space, so here are ideas that won't take up precious space.

As with bathrooms, suspending plants from the ceiling or on shelves is a perfect way to incorporate greenery into an office space. If they are placed in front of or near a window they create unpredictable movements in a breeze, a good source of NRSS (non-rhythmic sensory stimuli; see page 43). The natural motion of leaves swaying in the wind captures our attention and we momentarily take a glance, which helps reduce eyestrain and leaves us feeling restored.

Zamioculcas zamiifolia, commonly known as the ZZ plant, is an attractive, waxy-leafed plant widely recognized for being able to handle just about anything, including low light conditions. This means it's an ideal choice if you are a novice with houseplants, or your busy work schedule means you don't have the head space to care for them.

Fiddle-leaf figs and **philodendrons** grow tall and have plenty of leafy foliage, which are both great features if you find yourself distracted due to poor acoustics. They can create separation between you and the rest of the room, if you don't have a designated office, and can absorb some noise.

If you want something on your desktop, why not buy or make a glass terrarium filled with small tropical plants or **cacti** and **succulents** (they need different soil types and watering regimes, so it's best to stick to one type). Terrariums are self-contained and, if enclosed with a lid, can be self-sustaining, and need very little maintenance. These mini ecosystems are a joy to watch as they grow and develop and are a positive distraction on your desktop that can reduce stress.

> **Plants visible from workspaces have been found to:**
> • improve task performance by 10%
> • improve energy levels by 76%
> • improve reported happiness by 78%
> • improve reported health by 65%

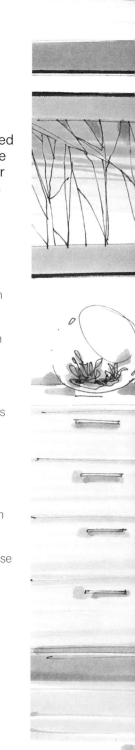

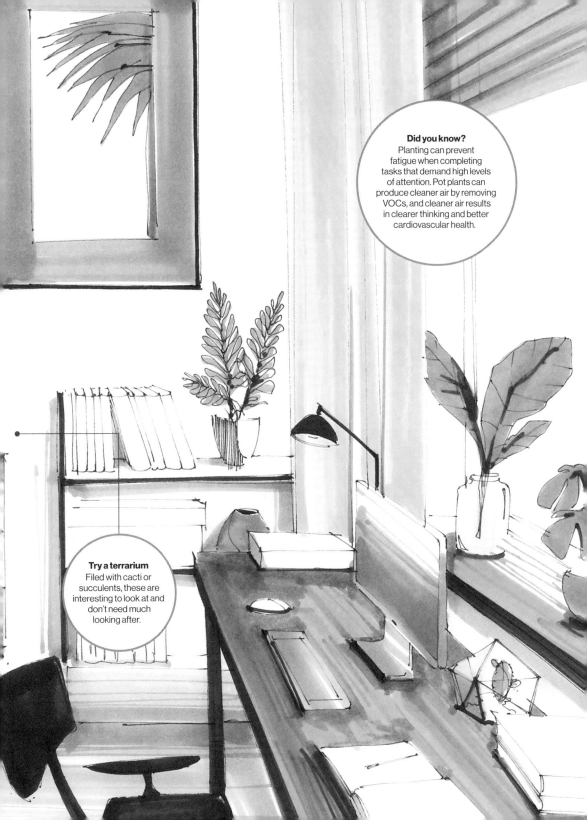

Did you know?
Planting can prevent fatigue when completing tasks that demand high levels of attention. Pot plants can produce cleaner air by removing VOCs, and cleaner air results in clearer thinking and better cardiovascular health.

Try a terrarium
Filed with cacti or succulents, these are interesting to look at and don't need much looking after.

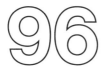

96 | Grow your own

A kitchen garden is an outdoor space set up to grow herbs, vegetables and fruit. It could be anything from a collection of fruit trees to tomatoes in pots, allotment-style planters, berry bushes or hanging baskets growing herbs.

Growing your own not only encourages you to eat delicious food that's full of nutrients, but also helps you stay active and increase your vitamin D exposure while you're outside. Did you know that time spent gardening also decreases your heart rate, promotes flexibility and strengthens the immune system?

Alongside these amazing health benefits, kitchen gardens can save you money and help protect the environment, since no harsh chemicals or pesticides need to be used.

> **Growing the plants that need extra care in the front garden, or close to the area you walk past daily, is a practical way to keep an eye on progress.**

They can also reduce your carbon footprint compared with shop-bought produce, since very little transportation is involved. This is especially true if you collect and swap seeds locally and use homemade compost, or join a community-composting scheme. It really is a win-win situation.

Position any high-maintenance plants closest to your home so you can easily access them. This could be vegetables that are at risk of pests, such as lettuce getting nibbled by slugs or broccoli eaten by caterpillars. Plants that are low maintenance, such as fruit bushes or trees, can sit further back, as these don't need as much care. Growing the plants that need extra care in the front garden, or close to the area you walk past daily, is a practical way to keep your eye on progress and a good reminder to water, prune and feed them. If you like being rewarded quickly, then think about planting fast-growing produce, such as perpetual spinach leaves or rocket.

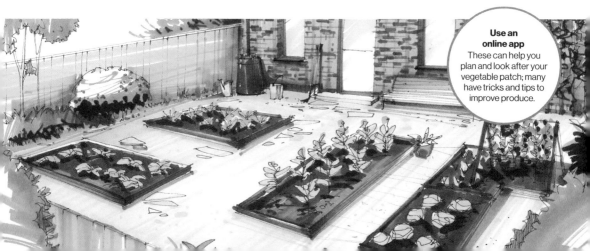

Use an online app
These can help you plan and look after your vegetable patch; many have tricks and tips to improve produce.

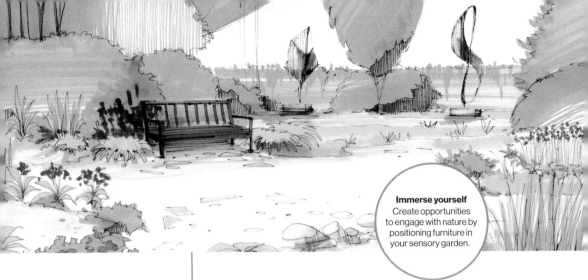

97 | Create a sensory garden

Sensory gardens are designed to awaken your senses: touch, scent, sight, hearing and taste. Time spent in them can be both calming and stimulating; you might run your hand through some tall grasses or breathe in the delicious smell of wildflowers. Giving yourself space for recuperation is vital for your wellbeing, to escape the pace and pressures of modern life. Here are some design features to consider when creating a sensory garden.

Our sense of smell is a powerful link to our memories, so consider planting flowers that remind you of a happy time or place. That way, when you brush past them you may recall those happy memories and find it easier to relax and reach a mindful state. If you can, plant a wildflower meadow, as this will encourage biodiversity: bees, butterflies and other insects will be attracted to the flowers, and birds will come to eat the insects. Before you know it, you'll have a thriving wildlife garden full of sights and sounds. Why not excite your taste buds by placing some edible plants in there too?

When choosing outdoor furniture to sit on and enjoy your garden, choose things that are highly textural, tactile and have symbolic references to nature. For example, you could invest in hand-carved timber stools, waney-edged benches or a rattan chair. For added playfulness, sandpits are a great addition to a sensory garden if you have small children. They encourage outdoor activity and can help us reconnect with natural materials. Sculptures and mirrors can also be incorporated to create a sense of wonder and intrigue, and to encourage creative thinking.

Don't forget about the acoustics
It's important to think about what noises you hear in your garden. If you're near a busy road, consider masking the traffic sound with wind chimes or the soothing sound of a trickling water feature.

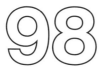

Make a mini garden

A carefully designed balcony can transform your day-to-day life. It can provide you with a space to soak in any available views, grow your own vegetables if you have no garden, and a place to simply sit back and unwind. Here are some ideas to help maximize the space you have available.

First, take time to check the orientation of your balcony, and whether it is shaded by obstructions such as other buildings. South-facing balconies with unobscured direct light may be too sunny for some plants, and it may be difficult to shade or move them. If your balcony is shady, use plants that thrive in low light, such as ferns, ivy, hydrangeas, fuchsias and Japanese forest grass.

Vertical planting is a great space-saving solution and adds thick, lush greenery that will be visible in your eyeline. You can buy domestic, low-maintenance green wall systems that can be fixed to walls to contain a dense variety of flowering plants or edibles. Or create your own with shelves filled with trailing plants – just make sure they're secured to a wall and won't get blown over.

Trellises can also be used to grow vertically and provide screening; plants can help soften hard railings and add pops of colour. Go for a type that allows light through, such as slatted or perforated wood, and remember to weatherproof it. Choose trailing or climbing plants that like to grow upwards or downwards, not outwards.

Many trees are happy to be planted in containers (restricting their roots will stop them growing too tall). They can be placed purposefully to create height variation, privacy from neighbours and shade from the sun. You might bring in olive, sweet bay, ficus or pine trees, which can be kept small in pots.

Another practical solution to save space is foldable furniture, such as stackable chairs or a set that can be packed away under a table.

Use mirrors to bounce light around
If your balcony lacks decoration, think about hanging mirrors. This will help create the illusion of more space and greenery, and will help bounce natural light – but be mindful not to create glare.

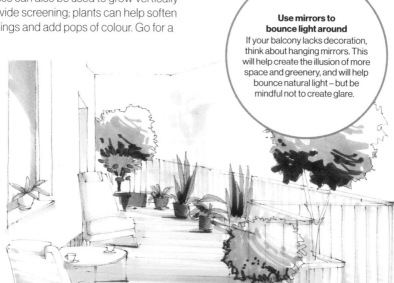

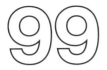

Cultivate a healthy microbiome

Biophilic design is an approach to design that aspires to reconnect us with natural systems to improve our health and wellbeing. As well as nature in the world around us, we also need to connect to the natural systems within us – our microbiomes.

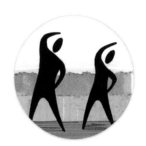

The human microbiome is a community of microbes (bacteria) that live both on and in our bodies, in our intestines and on our skin. In fact, the trillions of microbes that make up our microbiome can be found throughout our bodies.

The microbiome is often referred to as a "supporting organ" because of the role it plays in the functioning of the human body. Microbes stimulate the immune system, break down food and synthesize some vitamins and amino acids. They can be either helpful or harmful, and in a healthy body there is a balance of both. However, the microbiome can be thrown into dysbiosis (imbalance) by illness, poor diet or medications like antibiotics that can destroy the beneficial bacteria.

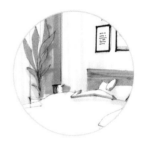

Scientific research has increasingly shown how important the human microbiome (often referred to as gut health) is for our physical and mental health; it has been linked to an improved immune system and ability to synthesize essential nutrients, and can also reduce anxiety and depression.

You're probably wondering how to cultivate a healthy microbiome at home. Well, reducing stress, taking regular exercise and good-quality sleep all help good gut health. We've seen how your home can support these things, such as removing barriers to exercise, enhancing sleep and using décor, sensory stimuli, layout and organization to reduce stress. Next, we'll look at how gardening can help.

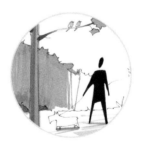

A strong microbiome is created through a varied diet that includes fermented foods and friendly bacteria as well as healthy fibres.

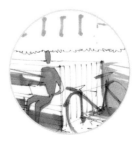

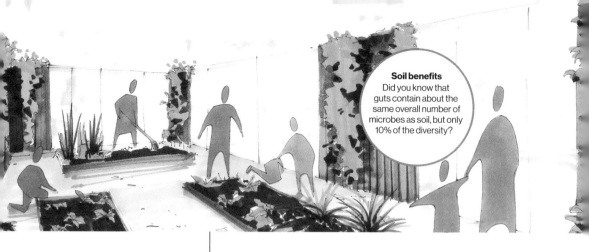

100 | Get your hands dirty

There is a strong connection between our gut and skin health, so it's important to remember the organisms on our skin and in our guts (the gut–skin axis) when we are trying to support a healthy microbiome.

A growing number of studies have shown that the microbiotas (communities of microbes) in our environments are important for our immune systems, and are looking at whether the more diverse and plentiful they are, the more resilient our immune systems will be. The microbiotas on the skin of young people have been found to correlate with local biodiversity – but the diversity of human microbiotas has decreased with modern urban living.

A study that compared the effects of children playing in gravel gardens versus mini-forests found that after a month the diversity of the microbiotas of children in the forest garden was one third higher than those in the gravel garden. What's more, blood samples revealed beneficial changes to their immune systems. The more biodiversity there is in our environments, the more diverse our microbiotas will be, and the better health we will be in.

At home, gardening is a great way to encourage biodiversity, and exposure to soil has its benefits too. There is a great deal of scientific interest in the benefits of exposure to microbes in soil. One beneficial type of bacteria called *Mycobacterium vaccae* has been found to be anti-inflammatory, to support the immune system and reduce stress. It seems that even short-term contact with plants and soil can lead to greater diversity of skin microbiota.

These are all great reasons to take up gardening! Growing your own food is also a good way to increase diversity in your diet by introducing different varieties of herbs, fruits and vegetables than those you might find in your local supermarket. You could also start fermenting food to diversify the types of microbes you are ingesting.

If you don't have a garden, look for local community allotments or gardens to get involved with. Failing that, re-potting and propagating pot plants and window boxes will give you a chance to get your hands in some dirt!

Further reading

Stephen R. Kellert and Edward O. Wilson, *The Biophilia Hypothesis* (1995)

Stephen R. Kellert, Judith H. Herwagen and Martin L. Mador, *Biophilic Design: The Theory, Science and Practice of Bringing Buildings to Life* (2008)

Stephen R. Kellert, *Nature by Design: The Practice of Biophilic Design* (2018)

Karen Haller, *The Little Book of Colour: How to Use the Psychology of Colour to Transform Your Life* (2019)

Patternity, *A New Way Of Seeing: The Inspirational Power Of Pattern* (2015)

Florence Williams, *The Nature Fix: Why Nature Makes Us Happier, Healthier, and More Creative* (2018)

Lia Leendertz, *The Almanac: A Seasonal Guide* (2021)

Tristan Gooley, *The Natural Navigator: The Rediscovered Art of Letting Nature Be Your Guide* (2010)

Richard Louv, *Last Child in the Woods: Saving Our Children from Nature-Deficit Disorder* (2006)

Dr Qing Li, *Shinrin-Yoku: The Art and Science of Forest Bathing* (2018)

Peter Wollehben, *The Hidden Life of Trees – What They Feel, How They Communicate: Discoveries From a Secret World* (2017)

Merlin Sheldrake, *Entangled Life: How Fungi Make Our Worlds, Change Our Minds and Shape Our Futures* (2020)

Matthew Walker, *Why We Sleep: The New Science of Sleep and Dreams (2018)*

Linda Geddes, *Chasing the Sun: The New Science of Sunlight and How it Shapes Our Bodies and Minds* (2019)

Tim Smedley, *Clearing the Air: The Beginning and End of Air Pollution* (2019)

Veronica Peerless, *How Not to Kill Your Houseplant: Survival Tips for the Horticulturally Challenged* (2017)

Martin Crawford, *Creating a Forest Garden: Working With Nature to Grow Edible Crops* (2010)

About the authors

Oliver Heath, Founder/Director of Oliver Heath Design
BA Hons (Architecture), Dip Arch (distinction) UCL Bartlett
My earliest experience of the wonder of architecture was on Brighton's old West pier – walking across the timber decking, delighting in the joy of the ornate penny arcades and the rush of the waves rolling beneath me. My passions for buildings and nature intertwined at this point, and I explored them further while studying architecture in Oxford and then London. In 1998 I set up my first design company and was picked to work in television as an onscreen designer and presenter. This gave me a platform to discuss the issues I felt were most important to the future of design: sustainability, for both people and planet. Since then, I have forged a path to bring the ideas of biophilic design into my own family life and to the centre of the design work that I so passionately believe in.

Victoria Jackson, Senior Sustainable Designer and Researcher
(MA Sustainable Design, PGCert Creative Arts Education, BA Fine Art)
I started my journey into biophilic design 15 years ago when I took on an allotment and realized I'd need help if I was going to grow anything other than weeds! A permaculture design course opened my eyes to the benefits of working with nature and how natural systems can be mimicked to design urban environments in which communities can thrive. I was hooked. As a practising artist and lecturer in art and design, I wanted to bring this ecological approach into my creative and teaching practices, so I studied sustainable design. During this time, I also set up the Brighton Repair Café, where people learn how to repair their things. At Oliver Heath Design, I continue to take inspiration from nature to encourage architects and designers to design for the wellbeing of people and the planet.

Eden Goode, Human-Centred Design Specialist
(BSc Psychology)
I have always been curious about people and what makes us feel and act the way we do, so I applied this curiosity to my studies and gained a degree in psychology. I left university keen to work towards enhancing health and wellbeing; I just hadn't quite found my 'niche'. By happy chance, I stumbled upon biophilic design, and it instantly felt to me like the missing piece of the puzzle. I now specialize in investigating and writing about the benefits of human-centred design, helping to spread the word about the importance of creating healthy, nature-inspired environments. I believe that by placing human needs at the heart of our decisions, we can make a real, positive difference to the daily lives of many.

Jo Baston, Designer
(BA Hons Interior Architecture and Design)
Born and bred in Kent, I spent much of my childhood building woodland dens with my brothers and exploring the nearby pebbly beaches. Since graduating in interior architecture and design from the University for the Creative Arts, I have been fortunate enough to work alongside some fantastic designers and makers. Outside the studio, my passion for sustainable materials led me to gain furniture-making qualifications and explore the beauty of natural timber. A highlight was assisting in the physical creation of timber-framed organic structures deep in the Dorset countryside as part of the Architectural Association's Hooke Park programme. These hands-on practical experiences inspire my design process and how I work with natural materials in interior design today.

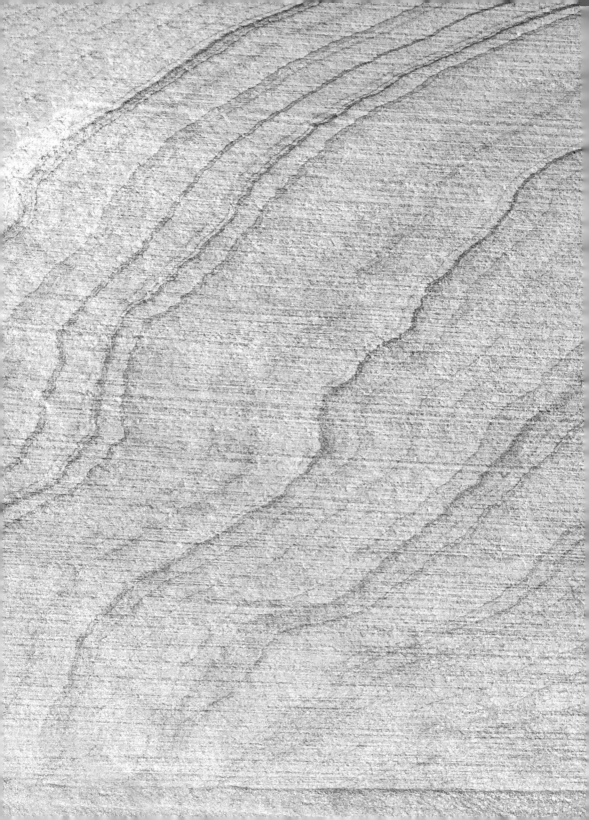